Racism and anti-racism in probation

Racism and anti-racism in probation analyses the complex processes through which black people are differentially treated by the probation service. Focusing on the use of *language* in probation practice, David Denney shows how subjective judgements made by probation officers can be given a quasi-scientific quality within the criminal justice system and are often used to justify sentencing practice. In particular, the underlying assumptions and perceptions of probation officers in relation to race are crucial in understanding the nature of the service offered to black offenders.

Drawing on ethnographical material and on his own wide experience of probation work, David Denney demonstrates how probation officers exercise power in a subjective manner, through judgements given verbally to the courts and in written reports. The process through which these are constructed and transmitted in a form acceptable to sentencers has a fictional quality, with clearly framed linguistic entrances, exits and interventions, all governed by a code of esoteric conventions unknown to the offender. All offenders are to some extent caught up in these processes, but Denney argues that black people are frequently unable or unwilling to be described and explained within the discourses of probation. He presents compelling evidence to suggest that some forms of probation practice can serve to discriminate against black people.

Through the analysis of this evidence and constructive criticism of current government policy, Denney is able to offer positive suggestions for improved probation practice with black offenders. He looks at the implications of recent changes in penal policy on the development of probation work with black people and considers anti-racist training and future practice developments in the light of current government thinking. His book will be specially valuable to probation officers in training, as well as to students of criminology, magistrates, lawyers, the police, and prison officers.

David Denney worked as a probation officer in Birmingham and London, and is now Senior Lecturer in Social Administration at the Roehampton Institute of Higher Education, London.

Racism and anti-racism in probation

David Denney

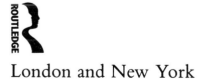

London and New York

First published in 1992
by Routledge
11 New Fetter Lane, London EC4P 4EE

Simultaneously published in the USA and Canada
by Routledge
a division of Routledge, Chapman and Hall, Inc.
29 West 35th Street, New York, NY 10001

© 1992 David Denney

Typeset in Bembo by
Falcon Typographic Art Ltd, Fife, Scotland
Printed and bound in Great Britain by
Mackays of Chatham PLC, Chatham, Kent

British Library Cataloguing in Publication Data
A catalogue record for this book is
available from the British Library

Library of Congress Cataloging in Publication Data
Denney, David.
  Racism and anti-racism in probation / David Denney.
  p. cm.
  Includes bibliographical references and index.
  1. Probation – England. 2. Discrimination in criminal
  justice administration – England. I. Title.
  HV9346.A5D46   1992
  364.6'3'0942 – dc20   92–2795

ISBN 0–415–06156–3
     0–415–06157–1 (pbk)

Contents

Tables and figures

Acknowledgements

A book such as this owes much to the collaboration and support of others. The research upon which it is based would not have been possible without the cooperation of Laketown Probation Service. Permission was sought and granted by the Chief Probation Officer of Laketown to publish these findings anonymously. Their understandable desire for anonymity means that the officers and those with whom they are working cannot be named individually, but I am grateful to each one of them for their openness and time.

I am also indebted to Brian Munday and Jean Hardy who in examining my Ph.D. thesis provided some useful comments which are incorporated in this book.

Mono Chakrabati, Margaret Dempsey, David Divine, Don Naik, Phil de Souza and other members of the National Steering Group on the Teaching of Race and Anti-Racism in the Personal Social Services have enabled me to believe that what I was attempting was worthwhile when my motivation was flagging.

John Eade, Steven Groarke and other colleagues at the Roehampton Institute listened and provided thoughtful help.

One of the major rewards that came from conducting this research was the opportunity to learn from Vic George, who was always available to offer analysis, advice and friendship. Such a brief acknowledgement cannot convey the international respect that Vic has earned for producing outstanding academic work that powerfully draws attention to human suffering.

Finally, I dedicate this book to Shirin Denney, who despite commitment to a demanding job has contributed her endless practical and intellectual energy.

With the help of all these people I have attempted to focus upon an aspect of the complex injustice that oppresses the daily lives of black people.

Responsibility for the final text is mine alone.

David Denney

November 1991

Introduction

This book examines the social construction of black pathology in relation to the probation service, an occupational group, working within the criminal justice system, who are statutorily charged to advise, assist and befriend the offending 'client'. Black people have raised fundamental questions about the legitimacy and purpose of the probation service. The answers that have emerged have wide-ranging significance for all those who are administrators and recipients of probation work.

Attention has been focused on black offenders for a number of reasons. Black people, particularly black youth, have been socially constructed as a problematic group. The popularised myth of a black threat is frequently presented as challenging the existing social order, as urban 'riots', perpetrated by recalcitrant criminals who disturb the law-abiding, peaceful country (Hall *et al*. 1978; Solomos 1988). This book focuses on the proposition that racism within the probation service may affect the social-work service delivered to black offenders, and concerns itself with three central questions:

1 What evidence exists to either support or reject the idea that racism or anti-racism exists in the probation service?
2 Is it possible to identify any differential processes operating in probation work with white and black offenders?
3 How do ideas about race and racism affect probation practice?

At the outset it should be acknowledged that the probation service is dominated by white people. In 1988, there were no black chief probation officers in post. Of the 250 assistant chief probation officers, two were black, while only eight of the 900 senior probation officers were black. Black probation officers only number 127 (1.9 per cent) of the 6,651 probation officers employed at all grades (NAPO 1989). In the main, white probation officers make judgements about black offenders.

Not just the probation service, but the entire criminal justice system is dominated by white people. There are two deputy recorders and one black judge in Britain. Black lawyers and magistrates are also notably absent from the courts (NACRO 1987). King and May found evidence of racism operating in the selection and appointment of magistrates within the Lord Chancellor's Advisory Committees (King and May, 1985). Consequently, black offenders face a criminal justice system which is dominated by white officialdom.

It would be an oversimplification to assert that the disproportionate representation of white professionals was the only explanation for discrimination against black people within the criminal justice system. In a recent review of the literature relating to the differential and discriminatory practices on the part of the police, the prison service, the judiciary, the crown prosecution service and the probation service, Reiner reaches the conclusion that:

> It is impossible to apportion with any certainty the contributions of racial discrimination and real offending patterns to the growing involvement of black people in the criminal justice system. It is suggested, however, that the most plausible interpretation is that both play a part, and furthermore that criminal justice system prejudice and discrimination on the one hand, and black crime on the other, reinforce and feed off one another in a vicious circle of amplification.
>
> (Reiner 1989: 17)

OPERATIONAL CONCEPTS

It is necessary at the outset to define a number of operational concepts which will be used throughout. Racism is defined as:

> The doctrine that the world's population is divisible into categories based on physical differences which are transmitted genetically. Invariably this leads to a conception that the categories can be ordered hierarchically, so that some elements of the world's population are superior to others.
>
> (Cashmore and Troyna 1983: 35)

Institutional racism can be seen as:

The policies of institutions that work to perpetuate racial ideol-
ogies, without acknowledging the fact. Such camouflaged
racism is not open and visible, but is concealed in the routine
practices and procedures of organisations such as industries,
political parties, and schools.

(Cashmore and Troyna 1983: 60)

Racialism on the other hand is described by Cashmore and Troyna
as:

The action of discriminating against particular others by using
the belief that they are racially different, and usually inferior. It
is the practical element of the race concept.

(Cashmore and Troyna 1983: 33)

The classification of human populations on the basis of racial 'types'
is impracticable, since no classificatory scheme yet devised has
been able to group populations into discrete categories without
ignoring inconvenient information. Biological differences between
human beings are relatively minor. No two human beings living
today are likely to be further apart than fiftieth cousins (Ely and
Denney 1987).

Cashmore and Troyna define an ethnic group as:

A number of people who perceive themselves to be in some way
united because of their sharing either a common background,
present position or future or a combination of these. The ethnic
group is subjectively defined in that it is what the group members
themselves feel to be important in defining them as united people
that marks them off, and not what others consider them to be.

(Cashmore and Troyna 1983: 12)

The word 'ethnic' is therefore also applicable to white English
people, although the term is more frequently Eurocentrically
used to denote blackness. An even greater difficulty involved
with the term 'ethnic minority' lies in the fact that it can serve
to marginalise and sanitise the ramifications of racism. When
describing the development of the race-relations industry some
ten years ago, Bourne describes the purpose of the 'ethnic school'
as being to demonstrate:

How these several ethnicities served to ameliorate, mediate,
buffer the injustices of white society.

(Bourne and Sivanandan 1980: 343)

Use of the word black throughout the book must be commented upon since it raises some important issues. In one of the research documents that will be referred to later (ILPAS 1982), the term black is commented upon as follows:

> The words 'black people' are used in this report when specifically referring to persons of Afro/Asian/Caribbean descent irrespective of country of birth, who consider themselves to be of such descent.
>
> (ILPAS 1982: 2)

Fevre points out that the word black has a deeper meaning than this in the British social formation:

> Some readers may complain that Asians are not black. Certainly research in this area is plagued by confusing language. 'Asians', for example, do not look like people born in Saigon or Tokyo. Nor are 'whites' the colour of this page nor 'blacks' the colour of print, but these terms have some use. They emphasise that to be recognised as non-white is to be treated differently to those with white skin'.
>
> (Fevre 1984: 9)

It is in the manner in which black people are distinctively identifiable and treated differently by white probation officers that the term black is being used.[1]

Many people in Britain are referred to by social workers as having a 'mixed racial' origin. In research referred to in this book, probation officers used terms like mixed race, and on occasions the more offensive description 'half-caste'. There is a strong view amongst many black social workers that social-work agencies should not distinguish between black and mixed-race people. Small has argued that the notion of 'mixed race' is misleading because it causes confusion, leading to the impression that 'mixed race' people are racially distinct from black people. This, he argues, prevents especially young people and children from developing a balanced racial identity. The term 'mixed race' is not given to the social worker by nature but created by the profession. Many black people find the term racist and insulting, denying the blackness of the individual (Small 1988). Consequently, the term will be avoided whenever possible in this book.

The term Afro-Caribbean is used when referring more specifically to those black people who define their origins in terms of both Africa and one or more of the Caribbean islands. This term should not be seen as the acknowledgement of an homogenous or national group, since cultural preferences vary widely between those of mainly African descent on different islands and between other ethnic groups within the islands.

Following the Criminal Justice Act 1991, social-enquiry reports which are referred to throughout this book, will become pre-sentence reports (PSRs). Although the probation officer will not make a recommendation in the pre-sentence report, she/he will still be required to provide explanatory accounts of unlawful behaviour including 'background circumstances', 'problems', 'motivation', and a description of 'attitude'. Much of the previous official guidance given relating to SERs will apply to the new PSRs (Home Office 1991b).

A NOTE ON THE STRUCTURE OF THE BOOK

Chapter 1 contains a detailed description of the previous research into white probation officer–black offender relations. Each of these pieces of research will be considered under headings relating to the methodological orientation of the study. The categorisations are referred to as quantitative, qualitative, and studies that utilise both these broad methodological orientations.

In Chapter 2 attention will be directed towards the way in which probation officers attempt to explain black and white offending. Chapter 3 provides an account of specific aspects of social-work practice with black and white people, while Chapter 4 will explore the significance of language in probation practice with black and white offenders. In Chapter 5, probation practice with black offenders will be located in a wider structural context, and it is concerned with the implications for black offenders of government proposals for changes in the probation service. The concluding Chapter 6 draws some tentative general conclusions relating to the possibility of an anti-racist form of probation practice.

Probation officers hold a pivotal position within the criminal justice system, exercising power in a peculiarly subjective manner, through judgements often given verbally to the courts and in written social-enquiry reports. Statements made in records may also affect the way in which other probation officers perceive offenders. The underlying assumptions and perceptions of probation officers in relation to 'race', will be crucial in understanding the nature of the service offered to black offenders.

Although previous research has been carried out in this area, it will be argued that little systematic attention has been given to the nature of the relationship between probation officers' perceptions of offending, probation practice, and the complex meanings that underline probation intervention with black and white offenders.

Race, racism and the probation service

In describing the existing research into probation officer–black offender relations, it is necessary to distinguish research which refers to probation practice and work which has been concerned with related but wider issues.[1] There is a growing literature on the sentencing of black people, which does not directly address social-work practice. Here, as with probation practice, a complex picture emerges, since a number of important studies seemed to indicate that there was little if any 'racial' discrimination at the sentencing stage of the criminal justice process (McConville and Baldwin 1982; Crowe and Cove 1984). Hudson, on the other hand, in a recent study of sentencing in London, found considerable disparity of sentencing for the most common offences like theft and burglary, commenting that:

> The vulnerability of the unemployed to custody, of black people to high tariff, very interventionist sentencing in run of the mill cases, and custody for even minor offences against the person, accompanied by the low use of probation for black males, was entirely consistent between courts.
>
> (Hudson 1989: 31)

Both Moxon (1988) and Hudson in their sentencing studies found a lower incidence of social-enquiry reports (SER) being presented on black offenders, which contributed to the low incidence of probation. This was partly attributed to the fact that black people were more likely to contest cases. When probation reports were presented to the courts, fewer probation orders resulted. Such findings lead towards a consideration of the probation process in detail. Much of the work in this latter area is relatively unsophisticated when compared with research into the workings of other parts of the

Table 1.1 To show previous literature and findings

Researcher	Date	Methodology	Finding	Explanation
Merseyside	1976	Unknown	Failure to make non-custodial recommendations.	Ethnocentric practice.
Ridley	1976	Qualitative	Over-representation of Rastafarians on caseloads.	None.
S.E. London Probation	1977	Quantitative	Over-representation of black offenders on caseloads.	None.
W. Yorkshire Probation	1978	Quantitative	Ditto.	Ditto.
Whitehouse	1980	Quantitative	Blacks under-represented in non-custodial supervision categories.	Possibly racism.
Taylor	1981	Quantitative	Over-representation of black offenders on caseloads at the heavier end of supervision.	None.
N.E. London	1981	Quantitative	Over-representation of black offenders on license.	None.
Carrington Denney	1982	Qualitative	Eurocentrism of white p.o.s leading to individualised assumptions about Rastafarians' licence.	White values dominate probation.
ILPAS	1982	Qualitative/ quantitative	Blacks more likely to receive non-custodial recommendation, but more likely to receive custodial sentence.	Possibly age or bias.
Gardiner	1982	Quantitative	Black offenders over-represented on caseload.	None.
Whitehouse	1983	Qualitative	White values dominate in SERs.	Racism.
Guest	1984	Quantitative	Structural disadvantage leads to over-representation of blacks in youth custody. No discrimination in courts.	Structural inequality.
Pinder	1984	Qualitative	Assertion of power by black offenders breaks down professional conventions.	Anti-racist practice. Power of black offenders.

De la Motta	1984	Qualitative	Whites more likely than blacks to receive non-custodial disposal. Blacks more likely than whites to have non-recommendation in SERs.	Inept practice.
West Midlands	1987	Qualitative	No differences in recommendations. Racist statements in SERs.	Racism of p.o.s. Racism in sentencing.
Mair	1986	Quantitative	No difference in SER recommendations. Blacks less likely to receive probation. Blacks more likely to receive community service. Greater likelihood of request for report on black defendant.	Unequal sentencing.
Green	1987	Qualitative	Colour blindness on part of p.o.s.	Racism in cjs.
Waters	1988	Qualitative/ quantitative	Race a 'marginal' issue in report-writing.	None.
Rogers	1989	Quantitative/ qualitative	Materials collected for monitoring purposes used by p.o.s in SERs. No attempt to consult black community in the planning of IT programmes and monitoring.	None.
Shallice and Gordon	1990	Quantitative	No difference in SER recommendations, despite differing histories.	Black people move up tariff due to p.o.s.

Notes:
1 The authors of individual pieces of research are quoted when known. In other cases the name of the probation area in which the research was carried out is used in column one.
2 Abbreviations used in this table:
cjs: criminal justice system
SER: social-enquiry report
p.o.: probation officer
IT: intermediate treatment

criminal justice system. The amount of data is limited, considering the complexities and importance of this area of probation practice. Although the quality of the research is generally marked by an absence of methodological vigour, an overall conclusion from the existing research is that black people are concentrated at the 'heavier' custodially related end of probation caseloads.

Such a phenomenon can no longer easily be ascribed simply to black pathology models adopted by white probation officers in social-enquiry reports, since, as will be shown, in the mid-1980s, some research has suggested that probation officers are as likely to make non-custodial recommendations for black offenders as they are for white.

The methodological approach adopted in the more recent research is difficult to characterise, combining both the qualitative and quantitative traditions. Despite the fact that there is no obvious historical continuity, it is possible to describe a number of distinct although overlapping periods in research development.

Quantitative research can be divided into an early phase characterised by the work of Ridley (1976), West Yorkshire Probation Service (1978), Whitehouse (1980), Taylor (1981), North East London Probation Service (1981) and Staplehurst (1983). The later work carried out in the positivist tradition can be seen in the research of Guest (1984) and Mair (1986). A qualitative approach was developed during the period 1982–7 by Carrington and Denney (1981), Whitehouse (1983), Pinder (1984) and Green (1987). Other findings appeared to combine elements of both qualitative and quantitative methods as reflected in the work of ILPAS (1982), De la Motta in Nottingham (1984), the West Midlands Probation Service (1987) and Rogers (1989).

Each of these pieces of research will be examined in chronological order, to emphasise the way in which the research developed over time. Table 1.1 summarises the main features of these findings.

FINDINGS OF QUANTITATIVE RESEARCH INTO PROBATION PRACTICE WITH BLACK OFFENDERS

The early quantitative period: 1980–3

The early work carried out in this area was initially dominated by local small-scale studies. The notion of 'small scale' is appropriate here since these early studies appear to rely solely upon the statistical representation of black offenders on the caseloads of probation officers in individual probation areas.

Husband noted that when the practice of Merseyside Probation Service was examined by the Home Office Inspectorate in relation to 'ethnic minorities', with particular reference to clients of West Indian origin, they were critical of the probation officer's social-enquiry reports, suggesting that more could be done to divert such offenders from custody. This group tended not to receive probation recommendations: 66 out of the 152 social-enquiry reports studied contained no recommendation. This suggested to Husband an ambivalence on the part of the report writers. When examining case notes the Home Office Inspectorate felt that clients were frequently treated as whites (Husband 1980).

Analysis of a caseload of city teams in Leicester in December 1980 revealed a total of 86 black and Asian clients; more than half the 'ethnic minority' clients were on the east team's caseload which constituted 20 per cent of the total for that team (Staplehurst 1983). The figures revealed that as a group, 'Afro-Caribbeans tended to be under-represented in non-custodial supervision; Asian and white clients had comparable rates to each other.

Similarly in Thornton Heath, Croydon, where the Afro-Caribbean population was estimated at 1 in 5 in 1977, a scan of the office caseloads revealed that Afro-Caribbeans were over-represented in statutory after-care supervision. 'Afro-Caribbeans' constituted some 16 per cent of probation cases and 34 per cent of cases in the statutory after-care sector (South East London Probation Service 1977). In a study of the Oxford Probation Service, out of a caseload of 300 in December 1981, black clients totalled 30: one 'Asian', three African, and the remaining 26 of 'Afro-Caribbean origin' (Gardiner 1982).

A similar picture was found in a caseload scan of Slough in 1976–7 (Ridley 1980), which revealed that the Rastafarian group of offenders made up 14 per cent of Slough's probation caseload, although the total 'Afro-Caribbean' population for the area was estimated at 2 per cent. In another caseload scan of young offenders in the north-east division of London, there was an overall ratio of 'Afro-Caribbeans' to white British of 1:2. In Hackney the ratio was even higher at almost 1:1 with the white British (North East London Probation Service 1981).

In May 1981, the West Midlands Probation and After Care Service and the Commission for Racial Equality jointly published the first major study of black offender–probation officer relations (Taylor 1981). Data was collected from standard statistical forms returned by probation officers to probation headquarters on a monthly basis. The purpose of these returns relates to the quantification of work carried out by probation officers.

The work showed that 13.9 per cent of clients were black. It is interesting to compare this figure with the estimated number of black people living in this country, which at the time the study was undertaken totalled 4.1 per cent. In addition to the statutory and voluntary sector much work was carried out in the preparation of social-enquiry reports, which was not researched.

The largest single group recorded as being in contact with the probation officers in the West Midlands were 'Afro-Caribbean', comprising 8.6 per cent of the total county caseload. What emerged most clearly from this research was the fact that black offenders were over-represented in the custody/postcustody category. If all licences are considered, 'ethnic-minority' groups were proportionately more likely to be subject to supervision on licence, following a custodial sentence, than the white group. Probation officers also had less contact with black offenders than white according to Taylor. When in prison, black offenders were less likely to be in receipt of pre-release help from probation officers. Taylor's work in the West Midlands indicated that 'Afro-Caribbeans' had larger proportions than their total numbers would warrant under children's supervision and on detention-centre licence, in borstal, as it was before 1982, or prison.

In the supervision categories (i.e. probation, children and young persons supervision, suspended sentence supervision, money-payment supervision and community service orders), all black offenders were under-represented when compared with the white group. On the other hand, white offenders were disproportionately over-represented in the non-custodial areas of supervision like probation, suspended sentence, supervision orders, or money-payment supervision orders.

In summary, Taylor's work demonstrated that although white offenders made up a majority of all clients, black offenders, particularly of 'Afro-Caribbean' origin, were disproportionately represented in the more punitive areas of probation supervision. The word punitive is used since these areas are more likely to be associated with custody, and in the case of detention centres, borstal and children's supervision, are more likely to involve the probation officer in 'recall' activities in which the probation officer is actively involved in proceedings designed to return the offender to the custodial institution because of 'bad behaviour'.

Whitehouse (1980) took one geographical area in the West Midlands with a disproportionately high number of 'Afro-Caribbean' offenders and carried out a similar counting exercise to that which had been attempted by Taylor. White and black offenders on probation caseloads in the Handsworth area were placed under categories of supervision, where another accentuated tilt towards 'coercive' probation contact was found. Only 7 per cent of black offenders were represented under the probation category as compared with 90 per cent for the white probation sample. The proportion of 'Asian' offenders on probation (1 per cent), was also significantly lower than recorded by Taylor for the whole county (26 per cent). Twice the proportion of 'Afro-Caribbeans' were found to be on detention-centre licence (14 per cent), at the coercive end of supervison, than there were on probation (7 per cent). An even higher proportion of 'Afro-Caribbean' offenders, some 20 per cent, were subject to borstal supervision. Thus the work of Whitehouse seemed to compound and reinforce the findings of Taylor.

The early quantitative studies pointed to the fact that young black offenders were more likely than white offenders to be concentrated within the custodial areas of probation work. This research also implied that probation officers might be instrumental within the discriminating process. Until the nature of the professional judgements which could disadvantage young black offenders was more fully understood, the significance of these over-representation figures would remain speculative.

It was also noteworthy that, with the exception of the 1976 Merseyside study, no attention had been given to social-enquiry reports. It was with the emergence of a qualitative approach to the research that a direct link between the over-representation of black offenders in non-custodial forms of supervision and forms of probation practice was made.

The later quantitative period: 1984–90

Guest (1984) undertook an extensive quantitative study of young offenders in youth custody, using data compiled from institutional records, social-enquiry reports and police reports. The research classified youths into three groups: black, white and Asian. For each of these groups, three longitudinal studies of social 'antecedents' and previous custody were undertaken. Guest found that the three groups shared remarkably similar histories of types of previous custody, notwithstanding the disproportionately high black population in the institution.

Guest found evidence of acute 'social disadvantage' in all groups, while the black group were more likely to have experienced what Guest called 'severe deprivation'. He argued that the likelihood of delinquency increases when children experience such extreme neglect and poverty. The criminal activity of the black inmates tended to begin during childhood. Guest did not attribute the high representation of black offenders in borstal to the work of the probation service.

Mair (1986) undertook research in two magistrates courts, which was intended to establish whether there were any differences in the way black defendants were referred for social-enquiry reports, the recommendations made by probation officers and the differences in sentencing decisions. Data was collected on all adult offenders, aged 17 plus, who appeared in Bradford and Leeds magistrates court over a specified period. A visual categorisation was carried out to establish what Mair refers to as the 'ethnic group'. The sample, numbering 1,173, was divided into black, white and Asian. Black offenders were more likely to be charged with offences connected with violence and drugs than white offenders, while Asians were less likely to have been involved in crimes of theft. No differences were found in the recommendations made by probation officers; and reports not containing specific recommendations were spread evenly.

Like Guest, Mair found that the average age of black offenders was lower than for white defendants. He suggests this could indicate that black people were being apprehended by the police at an earlier age than white defendants, or be a function of the age structure of the relevant populations. Mair's work also suggested that black defendants were less likely to be sentenced to probation, but more likely to receive community service orders, than white defendants. It should be remembered that community service is a high-tariff offence, which puts the offender at greater risk of a custodial sentence at any subsequent court appearance.

Shallice and Gordon (1990) carried out one of the most sophisticated quantitative monitoring studies of four London courts. Although this study examined a wide variety of issues concerning black people in the criminal justice system, including sentencing patterns, specific attention was directed towards social-enquiry reports and the workings of the probation service. This relatively large-scale study examined 578 black defendants, as compared with 124 black defendants in Mair's sample. They found that black people are more likely to be remanded for reports than white defendants. Although there was no difference in the recommendations being made by probation officers, similar recommendations were being made for people with different histories and degrees of previous involvement with the probation service. Black defendants were being moved up-tariff more quickly than white defendants as a result of the assessments being made by probation officers. Furthermore, this study suggested that report recommendations were more likely to be followed by courts when sentencing black defendants, since recommendations made in connection with white offenders frequently argued for more lenient treatment than the courts were prepared to give.

THE QUALITATIVE STUDIES: 1982–7

In 1981 Carrington and Denney undertook a qualitative study which specifically examined Rastafarian–probation officer relations. This small study was undertaken in Handsworth, West Midlands, which sought to examine an area with a high Afro-Caribbean population. Attention was directed towards the way in which probation officers perceived Rastafarianism and the methods of intervention currently employed by the probation officers in relation to Rastafarians. The personal responses of a group of Rastafarian offenders to probation was also examined. The sample consisted of a cross-section of 30 probation officers, including men and women, from basic grade to assistant chief probation officer. With the exception of one black male, the members of this group were white. A qualitative methodology was employed, based upon loosely structured interviews. The content of 15 social-enquiry reports on Rastafarians was also examined.

All probation officers interviewed found Rastafarians to be a problematic group, with a number of dominant conceptualisations emerging. The two major categories of Rastafari were referred to as: 'the true Rasta' and the 'untrue Rasta'. Respondents held that the true Rastas based their lifestyle upon a system of religious beliefs. These involved a number of rituals, including the smoking of ganja. This group was apparently more willing to accept probation intervention than the 'untrue Rasta'. The probation officers divided the latter group into two further sub-categories. One sub-category was often referred to as 'the Bandwagon Rastas' who were those who had adopted the outward appearance of the Rastafarians, but who, according to the probation officers interviewed, lacked any cognisance of the Rastafarian world view. The 'Bandwagon Rastas' were seen as especially vulnerable to manipulation by a second sub-category of 'untrue Rastas', who were perceived by the probation officers as a politically rather than religiously motivated group, with 'Marxist' leanings.

Causal explanations were offered for the Rastafarian phenomenon by the probation officers. Seventeen viewed it as an individual, psychologically determined phenomenon. Of these, some depicted the Rastas as facing an 'identity crisis' which had resulted from living in an 'alien' and 'hostile' society. Unable to cope and incapable of adjusting to life in Britain, the black youth, in a state of desperation and ontological insecurity, turned to Rastafarianism as a means of achieving a sense of 'self'.

Others advanced explanations which were reminiscent of Adorno's account of the authoritarian personality (Adorno *et al.* 1950). Probation officers alluded to the 'generation gap' to present a view of the Rastafari as an individual who, during adolescence, revolts against the strictures of an authoritarian father figure and a rigid upbringing based upon the ascetic values of the Pentecostal church. Paradoxically other probation officers attributed the 'Rastafarian's rejection' of the work ethic and values of the parent culture to the matriarchal structure of the West Indian family, by claiming that Rastafarianism stemmed directly from the absence of a strong father figure in primary socialisation.

The remainder of interviewees proposed 'sociological' rather than 'psychological' explanations of Rastafarianism. Eight saw it as a reaction by black youth against suppression – the 'unintentional stifling' of black culture in British society. The respondents did not relate suppression to racism. Only two of the probation officers interviewed perceived Rastafarianism as a sub-cultural response to racism. Although the three remaining interviewees did suggest that Rastafarianism may be considered as a reaction on the part of the black youth to their unequal position in employment, housing and education, none seemed willing to attribute these inequalities to racial discrimination.

Few of the social-enquiry reports made any reference to the Rastafarians' own stated beliefs. The reasons for this omission were never intimated. It was assumed that they were deliberate and intended to protect the client from the magistrate who was possibly unsympathetic to Rastas. In such cases the probation officer is placed in a 'Catch 22' position, for the social-enquiry report is meant to provide an unbiased account of both the social background of the offender and the background to the offence. If these reports are intended to provide the court with an understanding of the motives underlying an individual criminal act, then the failure of the probation officer to make any reference to the Rastafarian clients' beliefs must necessarily involve failure on the part of the court to understand the offender's motives.

All probation officers interviewed described problems in 'dealing with Rastafarians'. Lack of punctuality, uncooperative and some-times aggressive behaviour and the use of creole dialect were seen as obstacles to effective communication. The reaction of the Rastafarian to probation left many of the interviewees feeling cold and despondent. They saw their position as untenable and expressed surprise that so many Rastafarians were placed on probation. Most expressed pessimistic views when the issue of casework was raised, although some thought that this was an area where 'bridges might be built'. One third of the probation officers felt that black volunteers could assist in facilitating communication with Rastafarians, although some interviewees reported that they had tried working with volunteers, but without success. In many instances the respondents considered it more difficult for the black volunteer to intervene than the white probation officer.

Whitehouse (1983), while acknowledging the limitations of his own previous quantitative approach, carried out some important work which drew attention to the use of particular words in social-enquiry reports written on black offenders. The word 'ille-gitimate' frequently used in reports is for Whitehouse unnecessarily value-laden and unfavourable to the defendant. Often lone black women with children, supposedly living without male support, are described as being 'abandoned' by the fathers of the children. Report writers, according to Whitehouse, use conventional white cultural values to engender sympathy for women in courts, with the result that the men who have 'abandoned' women with children may be less favourably received in court.

There are cultural and economic factors which discourage stable partnerships. Rastafarian beliefs, argues Whitehouse, reject legal 'paper' marriages; and in a largely unemployed black community, income is maximised by both partners separately claiming state benefits. These important contingencies are not taken into consideration by probation officers when preparing reports for the court, according to Whitehouse. A consistent theme in reports examined by Whitehouse was the stability of parents. Those not conforming to a monogamous familial ideal did tend not to receive as positive a presentation to sentencers. Whitehouse argues that there is a tendency among white probation officers to 'learn a little more about other cultures', without examining the effects of their powerful white cultural assumptions which are included in social-enquiry reports.

Another important tendency emerging from Whitehouse's work is that most probation officers' explanations of black offending are given in terms of what may be broadly described as microsociology. Individuals, personalities, home circumstances and family structures usually form the basis of probation officers' explanations. They are generally wary of 'structural' explanations which take into account more abstract concepts such as racism, poverty and inequality.

When examples of structural inequalities are mentioned in reports, they are done so in terms that fail to define the nature of that experience. The following extract taken from a social-enquiry report describes the negative attitude of a black child to school. The child is described as being:

> Very susceptible to environmental influences. His own personality is fragmented. He has a strong awareness of racial prejudice. He has been reacting in negative fashion within the school and these attitudes appear to have coloured his view of life in general.
>
> (Whitehouse 1983: 48)

The mere repetition of these educational 'facts', argues Whitehouse, will create a less favourable picture of the defendant before the courts. Because the report is individualised, the failures of white institutions are frequently seen as failures of black individuals and will tend to disadvantage black people to a greater extent than if no such background information was available to the court.

In a number of publications Pinder has applied qualitative ethnographic techniques to the study of relations between black offenders and probation officers (Pinder 1982, 1984). His major study, published in October 1984, concentrated on the ways in which white probation officers 'make sense' of their work with black people. The specific objectives of the research were first to identify ways in which interactions between probation officers and black offenders could be handled more effectively; second, to identify the skills needed to practise in a multi-racial society; and third, to create a framework in which those skills might be developed most effectively.

Pinder used a combination of research techniques, his data being gathered from interviews with probation officers and an analysis of social-enquiry reports designed to identify ways in which probation workers assess black offenders. Unstructured interviews were also used in order to give probation officers the opportunity of elaborating more widely on their experiences in relation to black offenders. After matching selected white and black clients, Pinder undertook a detailed content analysis of elements which were seen as being central to the sentencing process, i.e. the terms in which the offender was described, the contextualisation of the offence and the form the recommendation had taken.

After collecting reports from 29 officers, they were then interviewed about their work with black offenders and the reports were examined with the probation officer. These interviews were transcribed and a copy of the transcript was sent to the officer involved. Pinder used a number of useful analytical concepts in his work. The notion of the ethnic/racial identifier was defined as a statement used to designate the specific ethnic/racial identity of an offender, whether by reference to origins, in the sense of place of birth, or by reference to experiences or qualities tied to ethnic/racial identity. Descriptions of offenders were defined as statements that served to 'assess' offenders in terms not only of their offending capacities but also of their social competence and personality.

Descriptions of offending behaviour were used to explain, or more accurately to contextualise, that behaviour and to relate it to an offender's life history and life chances. Assessments of the officer–offender relationship Pinder defined in terms of statements reflecting the balance of power in that relationship.

Professional conventions also emerged. These were described as statements implicitly or explicitly indicative of the assumptions which govern professional behaviour, and more particularly the relationship between officer and offender. It is the issue of whether or not professional conventions hold good in probation work with black offenders that is central to Pinder's analysis.

QUALITATIVE AND QUANTITATIVE TECHNIQUES 1982–7

The Inner London Probation Service published a report containing both qualitative and quantitative research material. It included a survey of all social-enquiry reports prepared by probation officers in inner London between 6 June and 10 October 1982. The survey also examined the subsequent sentence imposed, while an in-depth analysis of one in four of these reports was also included. On analysing the results, it was found that Afro-Caribbeans and offenders with one Afro-Caribbean parent were over-represented in this sample when compared with the total population: 15 per cent of the sample as opposed to 6.4 per cent of the inner London population as a whole according to the 1977 National Dwellings and Housing Survey.

It was also found that Afro-Caribbeans were more likely to receive recommendations for supervision at a rate of 35 per cent compared with 30 per cent of the total sample. Despite this, Afro-Caribbean offenders were more likely to receive custodial sentences in court, with some 26 per cent of Afro-Caribbeans receiving custody as compared with 19 per cent of the total.

The report also contained an account of a content analysis carried out by members of the working party conducting the research. A subjective content analysis of 100 social-enquiry reports was conducted, made up of 50 UK, white and 50 non-UK or born to non-UK parents. This sample was drawn from a cross-section of London probation offices. The purpose was to see if there were any differences between the service offered to clients from the 'ethnic minority' communities and that offered to white clients born in the UK. Reservations were also expressed as to the validity of qualitative research, since the content analysis was not 'scientific'.

Most reports included material and discussion about family background, early life, school, work, current lifestyle, mental health (where relevant), response to previous supervision and attitude to offence. It was considered that only 50 per cent dealt with these issues comprehensively and coherently. The other 50 per cent were at best not searching and at worst scant, giving the impression that the reporting officer had not fully understood the complexities of the offender's situation. A few reports concentrated 'very properly' on the client's current situation and a small number explained the client's attitudes and behaviour in terms of his cultural background.

Although there are a few glaring exceptions, most reports contained constructive and 'just' recommendations, with probation-service resources being utilised to a large extent. ILPAS comments:

> Clearly we are critical of the quality of a significant proportion of the reports, but in terms of service to the client we could find little difference between the two samples. If anything the non-UK sample fared marginally better than the UK sample.
>
> (ILPAS 1982: 35)

Having made this statement the authors went on to acknowledge that they did find examples of what they referred to as racial stereotyping and irrelevant references to race and colour, which could be construed as prejudicial, but no examples of blatant racism. The distinction being made here remained unclear (ILPAS 1982: 36).

In 1987 the West Midlands Probation and After Care Service carried out research which aimed to evaluate whether black defendants, when compared with white defendants, were discriminated against in social-enquiry reports. The sample collected consisted of 222 reports, 52 of which were on black and 168 on white defendants, and represented all reports presented at the Birmingham courts over a two-week period in March 1986. The main findings indicated that when black defendants were compared with white defendants they were more likely to receive an immediate or suspended custodial sentence: some 48 per cent of black defendants in contrast to 30 per cent of white. Black defendants were also less likely to receive a fine, probation, supervision or community-service order than white offenders. In this piece of research, unlike earlier studies, discrimination appeared to be located at the point of sentencing and not report-writing. Non-custodial recommendations were made in 90 per cent of social-enquiry reports written on black offenders and in 86 per cent of reports written on white defendants. Despite this, 57 per cent of recommendations on black offenders and 40 per cent of recommendations on white offenders were not followed. Where a custodial sentence was given, black defendants compared to white defendants were less likely to have had previous custodial experience.

Some 79 per cent of the burglaries committed by black people resulted in a custodial sentence compared to 25 per cent of burglaries committed by white offenders. It appears that the high incidence of custodial sentences for black defendants, compared to white defendants, could not be explained simply in terms of different levels of criminality. Black defendants appeared to be receiving custodial sentences for offences for which a white person was likely to receive a non-custodial disposal.

As well as comparing court outcome related to report recommendations, offences and previous convictions for black and white offenders, the research also examined the content of reports. This was with a view to determining whether black people were presented in ways which were overtly racist, culturally stereotypical or encouraged negative interpretations.

A simple check-list system was used to make this assessment, which required those analysing the reports to identify references to 'race', 'colour', 'nationality', 'stereotyping', 'value judgements', 'white culture', as the norm, client cooperation and the service's ability to assist. The assessors were then required to determine whether the existence of these factors was relevant to the report, harmful to the individual or reinforced existing prejudices.

Each report was analysed by two assessors to determine the level of internal consistency in interpretation. A sample of reports was then analysed independently by the research and information officer and race issues officer of the West Midlands Probation Service. Differences between reports written on black and on white clients were evident, with references to race/nationality/colour/country of origin referred to in 60 per cent of reports on black clients compared to 32 per cent of white. White 'culture' was said to be presented as the 'norm' in 10 per cent of reports on black clients, while racial 'stereotyping' was evident in over half the reports on black offenders. The researchers concluded that the check-list exercise had limited value in the absence of discussion within teams and guidance on the criteria for interpretation.

The selected reports were also subjected to an independent assessment. Examples of overt racism were rare but nonetheless noted in two of the sample reports on black people. One report written by a local social-services department on a juvenile contained the sentence:

X is a well built strong Afro-Caribbean teenager who has been
in trouble with the law for some time now.
(West Midlands 1987: 4)

The linking of racial identity with physical appearance and criminal
behaviour was considered to be a clear case of racial stereotyping,
presenting a negative image of no apparent relevance to the report.
The second report, written by a probation officer, concerned an
offence of physical assault following racial taunts and noted the:

Tendency for X to perceive himself as a victim of circumstances
rather than an author of his own fate. This becomes apparent
when X talks about racist episodes in his life.
(West Midlands 1987: 4)

The independent assessor noted that:

The report writer appears to put the blame for racist incidences
on the recipient by describing the client as being at fault.

No attempt was made in the report to present racism:

As a continuing feature in the lives of black people, nor any
condemnation of the racist incident which resulted in the offence.
Racism and its effects are reduced to an 'over-reaction' on the part
of the client.
(West Midlands 1987: 5)

Besides these two cases, there were features of nearly all the
reports sampled which, on balance, were thought by the authors
of the report to present black people in negative ways. This was
related to the style and content of the reports. By attempting to
describe clients 'objectively' (in terms of, for example, family
relationships, housing, education, employment), they effectively
created a description based on implicit assumptions of 'normality',
which failed to recognise cultural diversity or the consequences of
structural inequalities. For example, homelessness among young
black people was often described as a 'cultural reaction' to tensions
within the family rather than a manifestation of poor housing or
the necessity to leave home to seek work.

Similarly by describing family structures in which parents and
siblings have moved around the country, left home to find work, or
where children are looked after by brothers or sisters, an impression
of disunity is created. This can often lead to the premise in reports

that black people suffer from weak family units and that young black people are alienated from British society in part by the failure of the family unit to provide support. In any case it is questionable whether social history of this sort has any relevance to the offence, or recommendation, to justify inclusion in the report.

The unemployment status of clients was mentioned in nearly all the reports sampled. It was usually presented as a descriptive 'fact', with no mention of the disproportionate effect of unemployment on black youth. The report reader commented that without this structural context, unemployment can easily be perceived as a 'problem' of 'inadequate' individuals, particularly black individuals.

Contrary to Pinder's work the reader of reports found a high proportion of reports on black clients compared to white clients, where the mental state of the client was referred to directly, or in terms of 'abnormal' behaviour. This tended to be presented as an 'objective fact', without reference to any difficulties in identifying the nature of mental-health problems as they affect black people. Compared with white people they are more likely to be unemployed, to suffer from poor housing and to under-achieve in the education system. Moreover, client lifestyles which do not match ethnocentric definitions of 'normality' tended to engender negative interpretations. The authors of this report stressed that the findings of their research emphasised the care required in presenting information in the reports, while also focusing on the processes by which information is obtained, selected and interpreted.

A further independent analysis was undertaken of reports by the race issues officer in the West Midlands study. His overriding impression was that black clients' reports were treated less favourably than white clients' reports in the majority of cases, and, like reports written on all 'foreigners' and 'outsiders' which included Irish people, were written in a different way which was often unhelpful to the offender.

The poor structuring of arguments had a significantly damaging effect on reports written on black clients. The race issues officer noted that:

> There is a discriminatory practice of introducing nationality and the place of birth into the report, and sometimes colour, without any bearing or value to the case.
>
> (West Midlands 1987: 4)

In many reports on black people, the content of the report presented a negative image of the client where the same information could be reported more positively. The report writer's own values and experiences inevitably influence the way in which information is selected and interpreted. This can result in reports which are partial and potentially misleading when the report writer fails fully to comprehend and appreciate the client's social reality.

De la Motta examined 100 probation files relating to offenders between the ages of 12 and 14, half of whom were black. Her main findings were that first, a disproportionate number among her black sample had been charged with police assault, some 34 per cent if the charge of resisting arrest is included. Second, that probation officers tended to avoid the question of police assault in records and reports. Third, with regard to the inner-city disturbances of 1981, that sentences tended to become harsher for offenders involved in the inner-city disturbances of 1981, possibly because of adverse public opinion on the issue. Fourth, De la Motta contended that twice as many white as black offenders received supervision orders at their first and second court appearances, although she found no significant difference between the races in connection with the imposition of fines. De la Motta also reported that white offenders were beginning their criminal careers some two years earlier than blacks.

Like Guest, De la Motta describes most black offenders in her study as suffering material disadvantages such as homelessness at an earlier age than white offenders. In specifically examining the recommendations made by probation officers, De la Motta emphasises two important tendencies in probation practice. In her examination of social-enquiry reports she found that black offenders were over three times more likely to receive no specific recommendation in reports. However, the white offender was twice as likely to receive a recommendation for custody, although this occurred on few occasions – twice for blacks and five times for white offenders.

De la Motta analyses two distinctive styles of writing social-enquiry reports. There are, she argues, probation officers who make firm recommendations and those who do not. Fundamentally, the officers who fell into the former category attempted to create a context for the offence. In relation to the widespread urban disturbances of 1981, for instance, one officer described the feelings of insecurity and fear which permeated the area on a particular night. This contrasted with another writer who made no recommendations but simply stated that the outcome of the court hearing depended on the 'public interest' in this type of offence, i.e. public order offences.

In 1986 Waters undertook a study involving an analysis of 24 social-enquiry reports on black and Asian defendants, with the assistance of a 'multi-racial panel' who helped to score and classify all references to race, ethnicity and culture in reports on a positive and negative continuum. Waters convened the group, describing members as being knowledgeable about the criminal justice system, having varying experience of what he describes as 'ethnic' issues. The researcher describes the group as a miniature 'race awareness' course. After a discussion, each member was asked to discuss the references to race and ethnicity. Waters acknowledges that the end-product was a typology partly developed from the writer's own work on racism, social-work practice and ideal types (Denney 1983). Waters reached the conclusion that race was a 'marginal' factor in the writing of social-enquiry reports, not in the sense of a marginalised group or sub-class, but simply in the sense that 'race' was not a central issue.

A further study was carried out by the same researcher in 1987, where a sample of 41 social-enquiry reports were examined on Afro-Caribbean offenders. The rationale for selecting only this group was their over-representation on the caseload of the team being studied. The hypothesis for the second study was that Afro-Caribbeans would be placed in an 'alien category'. This would result in race being related to 'blameworthiness'. Waters describes an emergent equation thus: 'Being black + not belonging' or 'being black + not following the rules' and being 'alien' (Waters 1988: 90).

In this study Waters found that nearly half the reports made no reference whatsoever to race. Taken together, Waters concludes that racial marginality forms the dominant mode of report-writing. Waters goes on to conclude, however, that probation officers describe black offenders in a more positive light than is suggested by the work of Whitehouse (1983) and Pinder (1984). He writes:

> The high number of recommendations for probation oriented disposals, the concurrence rate between recommendations and outcome, and the obvious attempts by report writers to elicit sympathy are all indications of a more proactive approach by probation officers which does not accord with the notion that the courts or probation service are ambivalent or seek to exclude ethnic minorities from probation intervention.
>
> (Waters 1988: 92)

Green's work (1987) comprises a detailed study of some 138

court reports written on juveniles, and what he refers to as a close observation from the inside of the probation service's work with young offenders and in-depth interviews about race with 14 probation officers. The emphasis of this research was initially on the black offender, but eventually shifted to the probation service.

As part of Green's research, a 'survey' was made of social-enquiry reports prepared on juveniles in Wolverhampton. Green found supervision to be recommended by probation officers in only 6 per cent of black male juvenile cases. The equivalent figure for 'indigenous' male cases was 23 per cent. Moreover, the study also showed that while probation officers were less willing to commit themselves on whether the young blacks were likely to get into trouble again, where they did, they felt that it was more likely than with young whites. Despite this greater risk, probation officers were less likely to recommend long-term supervision even though the offences committed were similar. This resulted in black people moving up the sentencing tariff at a differentially rapid rate. Unlike the findings of Guest, Green's work suggested that black people stood a greater risk of receiving a custodial sentence (Guest 1984).

Rogers (1989) conducted a national postal survey of social services, probation and a selected number of voluntary organisations running community intermediate treatment, an alternative to custody programmes for juveniles. This data was supplemented by interviews with seven 'key people' who had a professional interest in the area. The aim of the study was to establish a 'national picture' of current practices in ethnic monitoring employment and training, as they related to the juvenile justice system. Some 91 per cent of social services departments, and 53.5 per cent of probation departments who responded were engaged in 'ethnic' monitoring. Rogers reported a response rate of 42.5 per cent for social services departments, 43.5 per cent for probation departments and 49 per cent for voluntary social work organisations.

Although most of the agencies were engaged in monitoring and anti-racist practices, Rogers describes considerable regional variation in the extent of monitoring and the use to which information gathered was used. Specifically she found that probation services used some of the material for social-enquiry report preparation, although the way in which such materials were utilised was not made specific. Good anti-racist practices as described by the author of the study appear to be restricted to the examination of literature on 'cultural stereotyping' and the development of anti-racist statements. Some work projects reported that they specifically addressed racism among juveniles as part of work sessions on the projects.

Significantly, Rogers found that voluntary organisations were more receptive to anti-racist initiatives than were the statutory agencies. There was also an inability or unwillingness on the part of programme organisers to involve the local black community in monitoring schemes and plans for activities on alternatives to custody programmes (Rogers 1989).

ASSESSING THE EVIDENCE

The studies described present complex and diverse accounts of the way in which young black offenders are treated within the probation service. The evidence varies in quality and quantity, as does the methodology utilised in these studies. The aim of this section is to examine more critically the methodologies used and the degrees of validity of the conclusions reached by these studies.

Quantitative studies

In the confidential Home Office report (1976) on the Merseyside Probation Service reported by both Staplehurst (1983) and Husband (1980), no indication is given as to the way in which evidence was collected. The only firm evidence offered is that 66 out of 152 reports examined on black offenders contained no recommendation for supervision of a non-custodial nature.

The evidence in this case is limited in scope, although this early report established a need for further investigation into the area. Studies carried out in Leicester (Leicester 1980, Staplehurst 1983), South East London (1977), Oxford in 1982 (Gardiner 1982) and Slough in 1977 (Ridley 1980) were equally vague in the accounts given of methodology. They merely represent the proportion of black offenders on caseloads at a particular point in time.

Other factors relating to age, cohort effect and geographical factors are not considered. More importantly, these studies can only suggest that probation practice is discriminatory. They tell us nothing of how racism or anti-racism may be operating within the probation service. Referring to these early studies Staplehurst comments:

> The unevenness of the statistics available provides very little scope for comparison. However, there are strong indications that the probation services' contact with West Indian youth is more likely to be in the form of coercive supervision than for whites . . . they are over-represented on caseloads generally, even when taking the age structure of the West Indian population into account. Rastafarians represent a particularly deviant group for unsubstantiated reasons.
>
> (Staplehurst 1983: 26)

The question of age is a crucial one and neither Staplehurst nor any of the other studies from which she quotes give anything like an adequate age breakdown. Since Staplehurst refers to her work as *Working with Young Afro-Caribbean Offenders* it can only be deduced that she has reason to believe that the figures quoted pertain to young offenders.

Another difficulty with these studies relates to the unclassified use of concepts. The Slough study (Ridley 1980) seeks to demonstrate that Rastafarian clients constitute 14 per cent of Slough's petty sessional division caseload, while the Afro-Caribbean population for the area was estimated at 2 per cent. The implication here is that Rastafarians as a client group are over-represented within the overall caseload in Slough. The problem with this assertion is that at no point is the concept of Rastafari defined. Another major weakness in the south-east London studies (South East London 1977) and those in Oxford, Slough, West Yorkshire and north-east London lies in the fact that the statistics are not broken down into forms of supervision, as they are in the Taylor, Whitehouse, and Waters studies. Simply giving percentages of black and white clients on probation explains very little.

What can be deduced from this cluster of small-scale studies is limited. It must be acknowledged that these studies, taken from a number of geographical areas across the country, point towards an over-representation of young black offenders on probation caseloads with a skew towards the custodial and post-custodial probation contact. This rather tentative conclusion fails to explain the nature of the interactions between offenders and probation officers which underlie discriminatory forms of social-work practice within the probation service and may be more relevant to the workings of the criminal justice system as a whole, and not merely probation practice. A limited statistical exercise of this nature fails to address issues connected with social-work practice.

Although most of what has been said about the earlier studies can be applied to Taylor (1981), it must be acknowledged that her work is far more extensive. The number of statistical comparisons are impressive, while her work painstakingly provides comparisons between the numbers of each ethnic group on probation officers' caseloads in relation to forms of supervision. Taylor recognises the limitations of her own work, admitting the work undertaken at the social-enquiry report stage needed to be included. She also argues that in 1979 the West Midlands Probation Service produced some 12,500 reports, which would have provided important additional research material.

Another notable exclusion from this work was discussion relating to the total proportions of black people living in each of the areas examined. What is provided is a rather inadequate statement from the West Midlands County Council household survey of 1976 showing that the total percentage of black residents for the West Midlands is 9.1 per cent. No indication is given as to the proportions of each ethnic/racial group. This statistical vagueness is marked in a study which is numerical in its orientation: it contrasts with the detailed description of probation caseloads.

A similar comment can be made in relation to other early quantitative studies. The studies of Leicester, South East London (1977) and the later Oxford work provide few details relating to the proportions of black people living in the areas studied, which serves to decontextualise research purporting to be quantitative.

Although we can discern certain trends relating to age from the type of supervision, for example in the case of children and young persons, some age breakdown would have added much to the quality of the statistical material, as would more detailed consideration of age and cohort effect.

The overall effect of these omissions is to decontextualise the early over-representation figures. Factors isolated by Taylor which needed to be considered in her study, as she acknowledges, include the age distribution of ethnic groups in the population, the composition of the white prison population and the nature of offences. Nonetheless Taylor's work, as the chief probation officer for the area argued, can be seen as an attempt to draw a baseline in a previously uncharted area.

It is in this manner that Taylor, and to a lesser extent the other studies of the late 1970s and early 1980s, should be viewed. They indicated that black offenders were disproportionately represented in the custodial 'heavier end' of probation supervision, although this discovery meant little without further elaboration and qualification. As presented collectively, these research endeavours raise more questions than they answer.

The research findings offered by Guest are of major significance since they diverge from the findings of the West Midlands study of 1987. The choice of Rochester Youth Custody Centre for research purposes is, as Guest argues, an important one, since it is a clearing centre for a wide catchment of southern England; findings based on this institution have wide implications for the whole country.

The number of offenders involved – some 4,876 offenders – is a significant figure. Guest also bases his study on detailed comparisons with figures for 'ethnic composition' for the south-east as a whole: statistical information notably absent from earlier research. He is able to provide convincing evidence of the over-representation of young blacks in the youth-custody system. Throughout the study, Guest also makes reference to age differences, which is helpful when he demonstrates such phenomena as the breakdown of homelessness at the time of the sentence.

Guest provides well-documented data to support his thesis. Most strikingly black and white offenders share much in common, particularly with regard to previous sentences, while greater numbers of black trainees were found in youth custody. This he argues:

> Is not attributable to inequitable court sentencing policies, but is more likely to be attributable to black youths' greater disposition to conditions of social disadvantage.
>
> (Guest 1984: 162)

A clear problem in the interpretation of the data emerges at this point. Black youths, according to Guest and De la Motta, do not receive custodial sentences at an earlier age. De la Motta claims, like the other studies, that young black offenders are more likely to be sentenced to custody and less likely to receive a non-custodial recommendation from a probation officer. The West Midlands Probation Service (1987) strongly suggests that black offenders begin their criminal careers earlier and receive custodial sentences at an earlier age, having served significantly similar proportions of earlier detention.

Mair's claim that he found 'no differences' in social-enquiry report recommendations needs further explanation. It is not sufficient to count the recommendations and non-recommendations for non-custodial disposal. It will be argued later that an apparently positive non-custodial recommendation can be worded in such a way as to make it a less attractive option to the courts. Shallice and Gordon (1990) introduce an important new dimension to the corpus of knowledge in this area. The suggestion that the relatively severe report recommendations on black people are more likely to be followed by sentencers could result in black defendants being moved up the sentencing tariff system more quickly than white defendants.

QUALITATIVE STUDIES

Qualitative work was necessary in order to establish whether the racism of probation officers and or sentencers was a factor which influenced practice, thus contributing to the apparent statistical tendency. This marked the development of more sophisticated forms of qualitative analysis and the emergence of studies which combined qualitative and quantitative research.

Whitehouse makes a number of observations from his work which are of salience to practice. He illustrates the confusion that white probation officers seem to experience when writing social-enquiry reports on black offenders. He is also right to point to the way in which probation officers appear to ignore or misunderstand the nature of the structural problems faced by black offenders. It would have been useful to have known whether such confusion also exists in the case of white offenders.

Pinder's work is remarkable for its wide parameters, its aim being to define and identify the ways in which the interactions between probation officers and ethnic-minority clients can be handled more effectively. Such an objective is general and overarching, requiring further clarification and focus.

Although Pinder separates the identification of skills needed for practice in a multi-racial society as being part of his reappraisal of social-work methods in this area, little attention is given to what constitutes social-work skill in the final research product. The body of 'knowledge' referred to generically as social-work theory is an important aspect of social-work training which could have influence in the shaping of practice skills. To ignore such ideas, no matter how critical we may be of them, is to ignore an important aspect of professional socialisation which could have a bearing on social work with black people.

Pinder's work is the most systematically designed and elaborate of all the studies so far considered. The qualitative methodology is clear and appropriate for the research task. It is designed to explore in depth the interactions between probation officers and black offenders. It is also a comparative study of white and black offenders which is a prerequisite for any meaningful assessment of the problem under review. Pinder quotes widely from his findings and is able to demonstrate his form of analysis with constant reference to the data.

Social-enquiry reports and transcribed interviews provide appro-priate data with which to attempt to understand the meanings that probation officers ascribe to their professional behaviour. Pinder's findings suggest an absence of an explicit framework for representing specific racial and ethnic identity in court, which is of great importance, and could possibly help to account for some of the over-representation studies of the late 1970s and early 1980s.

In short, Pinder provides well-argued and systematic evidence, albeit on a limited scale, to lend weight to the proposition that there is a qualitative difference between the way in which probation officers treat white and black clients.

QUALITATIVE/QUANTITATIVE RESEARCH

The ILPAS study of 1982 characterises this approach since it includes examples of both qualitative and quantitative methodol-ogy. Unfortunately the work contains little detail of methodological techniques.

Like the West Midlands study of 1987 which appeared some five years later, the ILPAS study indicated that young black offend-ers received more recommendations for supervision than white offenders, yet more 'West Indians' received custodial sentences. This important finding shifts the emphasis from the professional activities of the probation officer towards a consideration of the complex relationship between probation-officer recommendations in social-enquiry reports and the final outcome in court.

Another difficulty which is related to the lack of coherent

methodology is the absence of operational concepts. Words like 'culture' and 'racism' are thus used loosely and appear to lack meaning. In one case it is stated quite simply that in the opinion of the 'workshop' some of the material found in the research was 'racist'. Underlying the discussion within this report is the assumption that racism is so widely understood there is no reason to be specific about the meaning of the concept. As a result of this lack of clarity, explanatory criteria and categories seem to be confused and unclear.

Evidence is taken from a wide variety of professional sources, including hostels, prisons and community service. The amalgamation of ' professional accounts' raises a number of difficulties since the view of the probation officer in the prison situation will understandably differ from that of the prison officer in the field. Similar arguments can be applied to probation officers working in hostels.

In short, this would appear to be unreliable evidence for racist practice among probation officers, since it is often polemical, emotive and unsystematically collected and presented. The reader is not told how evidence was collected or analysed and the overall impression is one of unplanned randomness. The work also appears to lack a methological explanation which is an essential if the research claims to add to the understanding of differential service delivery.

The West Midlands study (1987) shifts the emphasis from recommendations and non-recommendations made by probation officers towards the sentencing process. Unlike the 1976 Merseyside study which simply suggested that recommendations for probation were being made less frequently in the case of black offenders than white, this study makes the unequivocal statement that despite the fact that the types of crime committed by black offenders who come into contact with the probation service are no more serious than those committed by whites, black offenders appear to be receiving heavier sentences. This study casts doubt upon the arguments of Whitehouse and of Husband who relate the non-recommendation phenomenon to white middle-class social-work values.

This part of the West Midlands work is corroborated by the London study of 1982. The qualitative work carried out by researchers in the West Midlands is more problematic and its inadequacy in this respect is acknowledged by the authors. The relatively high level of inconsistency between assessors points to some of the problems created by different interpretations of notions like 'value judgements' and 'stereotyping' contained in the check-list exercise employed in the West Midlands.

Any grid check-list imposes predefined definitions of situations upon the respondents when reading the social-enquiry report. Definitions on the grid are composed of highly problematic terms. In the first part of the grid, race, colour, nationality and country of origin are placed together. No explanation is given for placing them in this collective form. The placing of words like race and colour, and stereotyping in a check-list scheme, give the impression that objective meanings can be assumed, when common understandings in this area do not exist. This problem is acknowledged in the research findings and possibly contributed to the wildly differing interpretations of probation officers' explanations.

The research report required further elaboration, particularly with regard to the 'independent' qualitative assessments in which references are made to the effect of the poor structuring of arguments in social-enquiry reports having a differential effect on black clients. The meaning of poor structuring as opposed to good structuring is not made clear. Examples of 'stereotypical' expression also needed elaboration. In the case of the five social-enquiry reports which gave cause for concern, one single quotation illustrates the 'concern' and consequently the cause for concern remains implicit.

It was noted that a high proportion of reports on black offenders were described in terms of 'abnormal' behaviour in social-enquiry reports. On the surface this would seem to conflict with Pinder's finding that there was an absence of evidence of individual pathological ideology, conventionally found in reports on white offenders.

In his two studies Waters (1988) adopts a positivist methodological approach to his research. He takes Pinder and Whitehouse to task for theorising in advance of the empirical data and failing to give adequate attention to the quantitative data. He argues:

In research terms an adequate empirical study on race and social enquiry reports requires a large sample size well distributed geographically, so that generalisations can be made about different probation areas and different mixtures.

(Waters 1988: 87)

The assumption that bigger sample sizes can automatically lead to more valid materials in research is a highly contentious one and will be dealt with later in the book. Suffice to say that one of the most widely acclaimed contributions to sociology was made with a sample under 20 (Willis 1977).

Waters himself appears to be reporting on a study which had a number of important methodological flaws. First, the process whereby a group of knowledgeable individuals are called upon to make comments on a positive/negative continuum without commenting on how the panel was selected, and how the continuum was constructed, appears to be a highly subjective process for a researcher who claims to be concerned with positivistic purity. In 1988, when Waters was writing, in the light of widespread criticisms of the Eurocentric 'race-awareness' perspective prevalent in the 1970s, a more positive anti-racist perspective was developing. This appears to have escaped Waters, since he describes the panel in his study as being 'Like a race awareness course in miniature' (Waters 1988: 88). A similar lack of methodological positivism appears to be present in Waters' second 'replication' study in which 41 reports on Afro-Caribbeans was undertaken. This work, which is seen as confirming the 'marginality' of race in the report-writing process, lacks any comparative element and therefore must be treated with caution.

SOME COMPARATIVE CONCLUSIONS FROM THE EVIDENCE IN PREVIOUS RESEARCH

It is extremely difficult to draw any overall conclusion as to the validity of the research which has been described. Of the studies considered, five provided an ample methodological account: Taylor (1981), Pinder (1984), West Midlands Probation (1987), Waters (1988) and Shallice and Gordon (1990). Four of these studies, South East London (1977), Whitehouse (1980), Taylor (1981) and Waters (1988) provide detailed numerical breakdowns relating to categories of supervision. The question to be considered is whether the findings of Guest and De la Motta, when analysed, are different from the West Midlands survey (1987) and the corroborative findings of the 1982 ILPAS study. Guest's conclusion is based on the previous type of custodial experience undergone by black and white offenders, while the West Midlands study emanates from a close study of probation practice and court sentencing procedure, as does the work of De la Motta.

All four studies claim to have relevance to the way in which young blacks are treated in courts by probation officers. They reach contradictory conclusions, but this is not surprising when we consider the fact that they are looking at different research materials. There are a number of reasons for giving more credence to the work of De la Motta (1984), the work carried out in the West Midlands (1987), the ILPAS study (1982) and the research of Shallice and Gordon (1990) than to Guest.[2]

Having examined the previous sentences of young blacks and young whites, Guest finds consistent patterns of penal experience. Despite this, he finds a disproportionate number of young Afro-Caribbean offenders in the youth-custody system when compared with their numbers in the whole population. This contradiction is not satisfactorily resolved and points to the possibility that Guest drew a problematic conclusion from his research. The mere fact that black and white offenders share almost identical histories of punitive treatment does not explain the complex process occurring within the court, and interactions between probation officers, offenders and sentencers.

The evidence from the West Midlands study (1987) and the work of Shallice and Gordon (1990) addresses itself to the recommendations made by probation officers and acceptance or rejection of these suggestions by sentencers.

The West Midlands Study directs attention towards a number of processes in which probation officers play a part. According to this study, it cannot be argued that probation officers make fewer non-custodial recommendations in relation to black offenders. The evidence of racism was found in a small minority of the reports examined. Most of the evidence for this came from the qualitative work in the study (West Midlands 1987).

The West Midlands findings bear a remarkable similarity to Whitehouse's work in 1983, also carried out in the West Midlands area, which directs attention towards the selection of material included in social-enquiry reports and the way in which this selection process may affect sentencing outcome. While the use of custody is associated with current offence and previous convictions, there are a number of non-legal variables which could shift the balance from custody to a non-custodial alternative. For example, a defendant who is in work, lives in a stable family environment and has settled accommodation, may, all other things being equal, be more likely to be given a non-custodial sentence compared to a defendant who is unemployed, has a perceived 'deviant' lifestyle and is without settled accommodation. Black defendants are more likely than white defendants to be described in reports in the latter terms, which may go some way to explain the greater use of custody for black defendants.

SOME GENERAL EXPLANATIONS

One clear pattern emerging from the research so far described is the lack of explanation in the quantitative studies. Whitehouse in his 1980 study is an exception, suggesting that his findings point to discrimination within the probation recommendation and sentencing process. The link between the statistical data and this statement is not clear. Three qualitative studies, Merseyside (1976), Whitehouse (1983) and Green (1987), explain the differential treatment in relation to white value-laden assumptions made by probation officers. Pinder explains the differences he found in social-enquiry reports content in terms of attempts being made by probation officers to reach an authentic 'black' reality.

The studies encompassing both qualitative and quantitative methodology point to racism operating in an unintended manner, directing attention towards the meanings often unwittingly conveyed to sentencers by probation officers. Thus three general forms of explanation are offered to explain the existing research findings. These can be summarised as follows:

1 That probation officers perceive black offenders in a manner incorporating varying degrees of prejudice and racism, which constitutes discriminatory professional behaviour.
2 That probation officers, although aware and possibly anti-racist, are constrained by structures imposed by the courts, the wider criminal justice system and probation-service conventions, leading them to include some irrelevant information and exclude other relevant material from social-enquiry reports on young black offenders. Such practices can increase the possibility of a black offender receiving a custodial sentence.
3 Differences in the style of report-writing between black offenders are indicative of an attempt to present the reality of offending behaviour as perceived by the black offender. It is inevitable that in this process differences in presentation will become apparent

in social-enquiry reports. This tendency is linked to the insistence of black offenders on having their own view of their offending taken into consideration by probation officers. What is unclear from this research is the nature of the relationship between these explanations and actual practice.

Chapter 2

Explanations for offending

The perceptions of probation officers

In this chapter the occurrence of differing forms of explanation for black and white crime, as perceived by probation officers, will be considered. Initially, the main explanations for offending behaviour will be identified from original ethnographic research, collected by the author in a small town, which will be referred to fictitiously as Laketown. This research was carried out in 1987 over a six-month period. Social-enquiry reports on 50 offenders, 25 blacks and 25 white, were gathered from 13 white probation officers. The same officers were also interviewed in an unstructured manner (see Appendix). Explanations of offending behaviour from interviews, social-enquiry reports and probation records will be discussed in order to establish which forms of explanation predominate in each of the data sources. This will lead to the formulation of some general comparisons between explanations of offending behaviour for black and white offenders, as provided by probation officers. At this point it will be possible to identify the major categories of explanation for black and white crime which emerged from the research material. These will be considered separately with reference to the research material, in order to illustrate the qualitative differences which emerge between probation officers' perceptions of black and white offending.

The second practice section (Chapter 3) will examine a number of possible crucial variables relating to the differential treatment of black offenders. These include the acceptability of probation officers' recommendations to sentencers, the differing forms of recommendations between black and white defendants in social-enquiry reports, the differences between black and white assessments and proposed action plans, the comparative differences in aspects of day-to-day work and the differential forms of effectivity measurement.

FREQUENCY OF EXPLANATIONS FOR OFFENDING GIVEN IN THE FIRST INTERVIEWS

Table 2.1 indicates the frequency of explanations which occurred in the interviews with probation officers. Categories of explanation are recorded in the ways in which they were expressed by probation officers using their own terminology wherever possible. In Table 2.1, the traumatic family has been separated from other family-related difficulties like the notion of a disciplinarian father-figure or the mental illness of a relative. It can be seen that a total of 26 categories were introduced in the first interview (Table 2.1). The rates at which these explanations occurred in various forms in interviews was 27 for white offenders and 30 for black offenders.

The most frequently occurring single explanation for white offending was the use of alcohol, although if two family-related explanations are added together, for example, traumatic family background and marital problems collectively, they constitute the most popular form of explanation. Alcohol was only given as an explanation for offending in discussions about two black offenders.

The most frequent form of explanation offered to account for black offending in interviews was racism, which occurred on five occasions. In four interviews, probation officers mentioned 'anti-authority attitudes' as being a contributing factor in black offending behaviour.

Accounts based on similar 'anti-authority' explanations only occurred in one instance to account for white offending. Difficulties relating to the client's nuclear family accounted for white offending on five occasions in interview, while this was only considered to be an explanation for offending for two black offenders. Other forms of explanation relating to the family were given more explicit recognition by probation officers. A disciplinarian father and the severe mental illness of a relative were mentioned in the case of two black clients. The discovery of a daughter's lesbian relationship was mentioned in relation to one case of white offending.

EXPLANATIONS FOR BLACK AND WHITE OFFENDING IN SOCIAL-ENQUIRY REPORTS

Although the number of explanations emerging from social-enquiry reports were fewer than the number found in interviews – some 21 as compared with 26 in interviews – the occurrence of differing categories of explanation in social-enquiry reports was significantly higher. In the case of white offenders, explanations were utilised on 43 occasions, while 55 possible explanations were perceived by probation officers in relation to black offenders. The rate at which explanations were being used in social-enquiry reports was higher than for any other source of research data. In the following section which examines the qualitative differences in forms of explanation, it will be shown that in some social-enquiry reports writers used multiple forms of explanation, while in others explanations were absent.

It can be seen in Table 2.2 that the most frequent form of explanation in social-enquiry reports was the use of alcohol. This was slightly more prevalent in reports written on white offenders, with

Table 2.1 Explanations for offending behaviour

Interview 1 Explanation	White	Black
1 Alcohol	5	2
2 Traumatic family	5	2
3 Racism	0	5
4 Anti-authority attitude	0	4
5 Marital problems	3	0
6 Criminal influence	2	1
7 Sexual problems	0	2
8 Pragmatic offending	1	2
9 Unfeeling	1	0
10 Psychopathic	1	1
11 Incest	1	1
12 Lack of insight	1	1
13 Can't sustain work	1	1
14 Problem with violence	1	1
15 Victim of circumstance	1	0
16 Daughter/lesbian	1	0
17 Irresponsibility	1	0
18 Comes from a broken home	1	0
19 Would not accept stepmother	1	0
20 PO 'grassed on him'	0	1
21 Disciplinarian father-figure	0	1
22 Self-destructive personality	0	1
23 Mental illness of relative	0	1
24 Immaturity	0	1
25 Criminal reputation	0	1
26 Police harassment	0	1
TOTAL:	27	30

some ten reports using this as a form of explanation for offending as compared with eight reports written on black offenders. A traumatic family background accounted for nine white and six black offenders being before the courts.

The notion of irresponsibility was mentioned in five reports on black offenders, but was not seen as a form of explanation of crime in any report written on a white offender. Anti-authoritarianism was mentioned in some four reports written on black offenders, while this was not seen as a factor in any of the reports on white offenders. Twice the number of white offenders were 'led' into crime than were black offenders. Racism was mentioned on only two occasions when explaining crime in social-inquiry report, while it was mentioned on five occasions in interview.

OCCURRENCE OF EXPLANATIONS IN PART B RECORDS

These records are meant to provide an assessment of progress and tasks completed over a three-month period. Here fewer forms of

Table 2.2 Explanations for offending in social-enquiry reports

Explanation	White	Black
1 Alcohol related	10	8
2 Traumatic family	9	6
3 Irresponsibility	0	5
4 Anti-authoritarian	0	4
5 Provocation	1	3
6 Overcrowding	1	1
7 Led into crime	8	4
8 Instinctive criminality	0	1
9 Instinct to survive	0	1
10 Pragmatic offending	1	4
11 Depression	5	5
12 Reaction to specific event	2	2
13 Anger	1	3
14 Relationship problem with partner	0	1
15 No explanation given by offender	1	2
16 Sexual abuse as a child	1	0
17 Sterility	1	0
18 Racism	0	2
19 Unable to handle pressure	1	0
20 Mental subnormality	0	1
21 Authoritarian father-figure	1	1
Total:	43	55

explanation are given: less than a quarter of the number offered in social-enquiry reports. Alcohol was the most frequent form of explanation in records kept on both black and white offenders, although, as in the case with interviews and social-enquiry reports, this was mentioned on twice as many occasions in connection with white offenders than in records kept on black offenders. Problems related to the offender's family were mentioned in three records on black offenders and were mentioned on two occasions in part b records on white offenders. Criminal association was identified as an explanation in part b records on three black offenders, while it was not mentioned in part b records on white offenders (Table 2.3).

OCCURRENCE OF EXPLANATIONS IN PART C RECORDS

These documents record the contents of each meeting between offender and officer while keeping detailed accounts of telephone calls relating to the offender, or any significant event during the period of supervision. Alcohol was the most prevalent in explanations provided in relation to both white and black offenders, although it occurred with almost twice the frequency in part c records on white offenders than on black offenders. Racism was mentioned in three records on black clients. Explanations for

Table 2.3 Explanations for offending in part b records

Explanation	White	Black
1 Sexual abuse as a child	1	1
2 Relationship with partner	3	1
3 Emotional immaturity	2	1
4 Alcohol	7	4
5 Obsessional behaviour	1	1
6 Bad arrest by police	0	1
7 Refused interview at college	0	1
8 Lifestyle	0	3
9 Criminal associates	0	3
10 Little determination to stick at anything	0	1
11 Psychiatric problems	0	1
12 High lifestyle/low income	0	1
13 Family difficulties	3	2
Total:	17	21

offending were fewer in number and occurred with less frequency than in other sources of data.

With the exception of alcohol no form of explanation occurred with any notable frequency and the reasons underlying offending were often absent. These documents tended to relate to the daily interactions between probation officers and offenders and were more concerned with practice issues (Table 2.4).

SOME GENERAL OBSERVATIONS RELATING TO THE FREQUENCY OF EXPLANATIONS FOR BLACK AND WHITE OFFENDING

Table 2.5 indicates the frequency with which explanations for offending behaviour occurred with reference to the source of the data. Part c records produced the smallest number of explanations for offending, while interviews contained the greatest.

Table 2.4 Explanations for offending in part c records

Explanation	White	Black
1 Alcohol	7	4
2 Drugs	1	2
3 Physical disability	1	0
4 Relationship problems with partner	3	1
5 Inability to communicate	2	0
6 Rebellious behaviour	1	0
7 Obsessional behaviour	1	0
8 Sexually assaulted as a child	1	1
9 Acting out being a criminal	0	1
10 Racism	0	3
11 Anger	0	1
12 Offends to get money fast	0	1
13 Mother incapable of exerting authority	0	1
14 Refused interview at college	0	1
Total:	17	16

Social-enquiry reports followed close behind interviews when the number of different explanations were examined. Explanations occur with the greatest frequency in social-enquiry reports on black offenders. Explanations of white offending were most frequently expressed in social-enquiry reports. Interviews provided the next greatest frequency of explanations although, as was the case with social-enquiry reports, more explanations were offered with greater frequency in the case of black than white offenders. There was little notable difference between the frequencies of explanation offered in part c and b records, although there was slightly lower frequency in part c than b records. Throughout the material, explanations of black crime occurred with greater frequency than did explanations of white crime.

Explanations of black crime were more likely to be expressed in social-enquiry reports on black offenders than they were in social-enquiry reports on white offenders. Probation officers, however, were less likely to offer explanations of black offending in interviews than they were of white offending. In part b records, one of the most obvious incongruities occurred between the frequency with which explanations were offered in the case of black and white offenders. Almost twice the number of explanations were given in part c records on black offenders than on white offenders. The frequency with which explanations were given in part c records were fairly consistent for black and white offenders.

Table 2.6 represents a breakdown of the major forms of explanation for offending which emerged from all sources of data. For the purposes of this book, 'major' refers to explanations occurring on three or more occasions in each separate source of data.

The most prevalent form of explanation of crime for black and white offenders was the use of alcohol, although this occurred with greater frequency in relation to white offenders. Probation officers identified 'family problems' as contributing to offending behaviour in a relatively high proportion of black and white 'cases'. Family

Table 2.5 To show comparative frequency of explanations for offending

Source of explanation	Number of different explanations for black and white	White	Black
		Frequency	
Part c records	14	17	16
Part b records	13	18	20
Interview 1	26	27	30
30 SERs	21	43	54

problems were more likely to be identified as being significant for white offenders. Anti-authoritarianism emerged as an all-black phenomenon in this research.

Racism was the next most prevalent explanation which occurred on seven occasions. Twice the number of white offenders were perceived to be led into crime in social-enquiry reports than were

Table 2.6 To show the number of explanations for offending behaviour occurring three or more times for black and white subjects

Interview 1	
White	
Alcohol	5
Family-related factors	5
Relationship/marital problems	3
Black	
Racism	5
Social-enquiry reports	
White	
Alcohol	10
Family	10
Led into crime	8
Depression	4
Black	
Alcohol	8
Family	10
Irresponsibility	5
Anti-authoritarianism	4
Provocation	3
Led into crime	4
Pragmatic offending	4
Anger	3
Part b records	
White	
Alcohol	4
Lifestyle	3
Criminal associates	3
Alcohol	7
Relationship with partner	3
Family difficulties	3
Part c records	
White	
Alcohol	7
Relationship problems	3
Black	
Alcohol	4
Acting out being a criminal	3

black offenders. In part b records, three offenders were seen by probation officers as being influenced by criminal associates. Relationship problems were more evenly spread between black and white offenders when part c and b records were examined. In social-enquiry reports, a significant number of black offenders were seen as being provoked into crime.

Pragmatic offending occurred with a significant frequency in social-enquiry reports on black offenders. Anger, an apparently black phenomenon, again occurred with most frequency in social-enquiry reports. The influence of 'lifestyle' was mentioned on one occasion in a part b record on a black offender. The effect of problems emanating from difficulties in relationships, although more evenly spread among accounts given of black and white offending, appeared with most regularity in connection with white offenders during interviews. Here marital relationships were specifically identified as having a possible influence on offending. In part b records, problems with relationships were seen as having a significant effect on criminal behaviour for black clients.

When probation officers attempted to explain black and white crime in social-enquiry reports, a number of explanations dominate. For both black and white offenders the use of alcohol and accounts related to the family dominate. Racism and behaviour which is seen as encompassing anti-authoritarian sentiment dominate in explanations given of black offending. The manner in which these explanations are presented in various sources will now be examined.

OFFENDING AND THE USE OF ALCOHOL

The use of alcohol was by far the most dominant explanation given for black and white offending in all sources of data. The idea that alcohol is a problem which could have an influence on offending seems to be presented as a matter of fact: little effort is made to explain the nature of the connection. In a social-enquiry report on a black offender relating to an offence of actual bodily harm, the probation officer writes:

> I asked him about his drinking. Although his overall consumption of alcohol seems to be within safe limits, on a night out he will drink heavily. This would seem to be directly connected with his offending.

In this report, as in the case with most social-enquiry reports in which drink was cited as an explanatory factor in the commission of crime, alcohol was not the principal cause of crime, since a differentiated form of explanation was provided. Alcohol was frequently conceptualised in terms of being a factor which 'triggered offending', as the following extract from a social-enquiry report concerning a black offender illustrates:

> He had drunk a beer and at least one measure of spirits at lunch time, and began drinking heavily again at about X p.m. By the time he arrived at the pub he was intoxicated, and he then had three cans of extra strong lager and four further bottles of beer (at least, because his memory is cloudy). Mr X (the defendant) said that the victim of the offence was probably a little drunk herself, and was going around the pub asking for a Christmas kiss. Mr X said that he refused, and a little later he says that he accidentally brushed into the girl, who swore at him for not giving her a kiss. An argument developed during which he was called a 'black bastard' and he lost control.

The subject of the report then attacked the girl, which resulted in his being charged with actual bodily harm. The interactions immediately preceding suggest that the offender was the victim of racial abuse. The consumption of alcohol then triggered the offending behaviour. This sequence of events is then contrasted with the 'real' underlying cause of the incident as seen by the probation officer, which in this case is clearly expressed later in the report:

> It is note worthy that the assault last year (referring to a similar offence) was also on a woman, and it is plausible that he projects his hostility towards his mother, on to women in general.

Thus in this case both alcohol and the argument which developed in the public house resulting in the defendant being called a black bastard take second place to the notion of the offender projecting his hostility towards his mother and on women in general. This assertion is made without any reference or evidence in the report to support it.

In this report, even though the officer uses the words constituting the racial insult to great effect, the underlying explanation is based on speculative comments connected with the offender's use of alcohol and the projection of hostile feelings towards his mother and women. The combination of alcohol, a safe, conventional form of explanation, and a quasi-psychoanalytic statement take clear explanatory precedence over a direct and reported racial insult. Such a tendency was also noted in the work carried out by the West Midlands Probation Service in 1987, in which report-writers noted the reluctance to explain offending behaviour directly in terms of a response to racist insults or attacks. The projection of negative feelings towards the defendant's mother also represents an attempt to explain the oppressive nature of a male attack on a woman. Such highly individualised explanations indicate a reluctance to approach racism or the oppression of women in social-enquiry reports.

In cases in which the black offender's use of alcohol was used as a factor in explaining crime, drinking was described in terms of 'sparking off' a situation in which the offender ultimately participated. In the latter case this was the social situation in which the offender found himself. There was no intimation that the use of alcohol could singularly be regarded as a cause of offending.

A similar observation can be made of the way in which the use of alcohol is described in social-enquiry reports on young white offenders as the following extract from a report indicates:

> From what Mr X has told me it appears that he and his wife have a stormy relationship which worsens when they have been drinking.

In the same social-enquiry report, drink is related to burglary when the writer of the report describes the offender's drinking as a partial explanation for the offence:

> Mr X tells me that he did not think of the consequences of committing the offences, and it appears that this is the normal pattern of behaviour whereby he acts first, and thinks about what he has done after the event. It also appears that the offences occurred when the defendant had been drinking.

Here the problem is located within the individual, in that he thinks after he has acted: a feature of his personality worsened by drink. Like the black offender, there was a temporary lapse of thought and loss of control which accounted for the offending behaviour. It is implicit that had the offender followed his usual pattern of thinking, the offence would not have occurred.

It is also possible for the probation officer to use the 'kicking'

of alcohol as a factor in favour of the defendant, as we see in the
following extract from a social-enquiry report:

> In the past his drinking was excessive, indeed it was associated
> with earlier offending, but this is no longer the case. Alcohol is
> not drunk in the house and visits to the pub are limited to once
> a week.

Here the writer makes reference to the stability of family life as
being an indication of the tendency towards 'reformation'.

Reformation and the conquering of alcohol was an almost
exclusively white phenomenon in this research. It was mentioned
in five reports on white offenders in which alcohol was emphasised
as a principal cause of offending. Alcohol was used frequently in
interviews as an explanation for offending and it was mentioned
by probation officers without being prompted. In one interview
the following interchange took place when discussing a black
offender:

> DD: How do you think X got himself into the position
> he is in?
> PO: Essentially what happened is that he had had too much
> to drink on Christmas Eve, and he hit somebody, that's
> the short answer.

Indeed, 'short answers' seemed to be given in relation to the
likely effect of alcohol on black offending while explanations
were more forthcoming in relation to white offenders' drinking.
The same probation officer, when describing a white client in an
interview, said:

> From being a young teenage tearaway he has turned into an
> adult who is settled down. He has a couple of children and a
> very good work record, he has a very high earning capacity,
> and he has made a jump from spending a lot of time with his
> mates in the boozer to a more home-centred life. He spends far
> less time with mates in the boozer, but even now these episodes
> do represent a high risk for him, and he is likely when at risk to
> find himself back in trouble, but he has changed. I have known
> him for a couple of years and he has worked very hard.

Here the transformation of the 'tearaway' into a responsible adult
was evidenced by performance indicators which were frequently

used in describing the white offender's metamorphosis: a process which did not appear in accounts given of black offenders. The offender described above had 'settled down' in that he had a family, a good work record and a more 'home-centred life'. The only risk was seen as alcohol, which had also for the most part been brought under control.

Although the use of alcohol was mentioned in the interview without prompting in relation to white offenders, probation officers were not anxious to develop the topic in any detail when discussing black offending behaviour.

In part c records on black and white offenders, drinking was rarely mentioned. This could well have been accounted for by the fact that over 70 per cent of the defendants who had been described in social-enquiry reports as having a drink-related problem had been referred to a special alcohol-centred group, where separate records were kept. Similarly in part b records on black offenders, very little reference was made to alcohol, although slightly more reference was made to problems relating to alcohol in part b records written on white offenders. There would seem to be little to account for this finding, except that it may reflect a reluctance on the part of probation officers to reflect in detail on this explanation of offending-related behaviour in a written form.

The stereotypical macho male was associated with drink – and a particular brand of drink, as can be seen in the following part b record on a white offender:

> The prognosis on X is poor, and there is a good chance that he will go into youth custody. The main task is to get the probation order alive as he is aware that he may go down and therefore has little interest. There are areas to be tackled with an obvious emphasis on his offending which seems to stem from his carefree attitude, his sometimes excessive alcohol consumption, and his relationship with his male peers, which is fundamentally different from his relationship with his girlfriend. He is very much into the stereotypical macho image, I bet he drinks Carling black label.

Such a stereotype was not present in any of the material relating to drink, or any other matter connected with black offending. It is noteworthy that probation officers felt able to represent white offenders officially in terms of white populist images.

The same probation officer in an initial assessment on another white offender describes the drink factor contributing to the offender's criminal activities in a manner which characterised many probation officers' views of white crime causation:

> X appears to be highly motivated in his attempts to keep out of trouble, his offending would appear to be stress, and probably drink related, his relationship with his wife is very important, although I believe she creates a pressure for him, because she is so dependant on X.

A highly stressed young man is being presented here whose wife seems to create a further burden. He is described by the probation officer in very positive terms as being 'highly motivated' as he attempts to keep out of trouble, while drink is presented as a likely factor in offending. The reference to drink is placed between the references to stress and his wife, as is shown figuratively below.

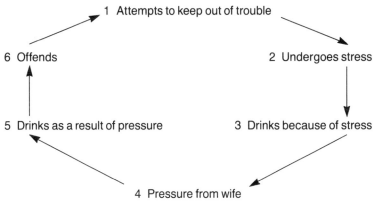

Figure 2.1   To show cyclical form of explanation in relation to white crime

Here a cyclical explanation is given, which presented itself on eight occasions with slight variations, to account for white crime. Such generalised perceptions of causation were not present in explanations of black crime. This observation lends weight to some extent to the work of Pinder (1984) who found explanations of black crime to be more individualised and unconventional. These findings differ from Pinder's work in that the notion of the victim occurs in reports on black and white offenders. This concept also effectively explains offending in terms of events external to the offender being beyond her/his control. These factors are not connected to individual pathology, which is 'punishable' by the court. Both the Carling image and that of the stressed drinker present the offender as a victim. The first is a victim of advertising with the resultant connotative aspirations and consumption of the product Carling Black Label.

The second is a victim of stress caught in the cycle of drink-related offending shown in Figure 2.1. This is significant since the process of offending described in relation to the black client seems unconventional and frivolous. The officer seems to be struggling to provide a coherent explanation, while the account given of white offending follows a conventional pattern which would have a reasonable chance of being acceptable to the courts. Such a phenomenon is further exemplified in the following extract from a part c record which refers to a white disabled offender:

> It is clear that his resentment, and sadness for the past has undermined his self confidence. In our interview he linked his offending to feelings of anger, sometimes exacerbated by drinking, there were certain key incidents connected with his brother, and with the disabled label he was given, which seemed to trigger this anger off.

Here we see the complex juxtaposition of words, the effect of which is to make the unacceptable acceptable. 'Resentment', a term with negative connotations, is tempered by sadness, while anger, another negative term, does not reflect the nature of the personality involved, since his anger is partly created by drinking. Specific incidents concerning his brother have further exacerbated the situation to create a criminal reaction. The effects of these factors are then combined with the disabled label, which finally triggers off the offending behaviour. The use of contrasting words serves to diminish an alternative impression, which could have been presented, of a disabled person who has problems controlling his anger in certain situations of stress.

The important point emerging from the study of explanations based on alcohol is that its popularity among probation officers is indicative of a need to present an explanation of behaviour which is acceptable to the courts and can indeed make the offender appear to be a victim. This applies equally to white and black offenders. The qualitative difference lies in the fact that the form of explanation given in relation to white offenders follows a conventional pattern which is relatable to the cultural experience of the white probation officer, magistrate and judge, while the alternative and highly individualised form of explanation given of black offending lacks a coherent form or convention. There is in Pinder's words an absence of a 'coherent and explicit framework' in representing black crime.

OFFENDING AND THE FAMILY

Probation officers used explanations for offending based on difficulties generated within the black family with considerable frequency. The material presented here seeks to demonstrate that probation officers appeared to express confusion as to the meanings that black people ascribe to family life. Probation officers generally showed a tendency to attempt to impose a white anglicised view of the nuclear family when making statements and judgements about black families. This frequently resulted in the creation of stereotypical images.

The process described here appears to operate at a number of levels. At the implicit level the probation officer makes conceptual linkages which lead the reader to certain conclusions about family life. In X's social-enquiry report offending was explained in the following manner:

> X is one of five children. The records indicated a turbulent, and violent home background. His mother died when he was three, and his father subsequently married three times. His marriage has been characterised by disharmony and violence from his father. His father is a heavy drinker, which apparently aggravates his temper. Predictably, therefore, the children spent periods in care. Perhaps this violent background goes some way to explaining the number of offences of aggression.

Here there is a link made between the subject's offending, a large family, his mother's death and his father's subsequent marriages and cruelty. The authoritarian father-figure appeared in a number of social-enquiry reports and black parenting was often seen as being directly related to crime. Here, as in many accounts of black family life, the aggression experienced by the offender at home is linked to the aggression displayed in criminal activities. This connection was far more clearly defined and more prevalent in accounts of black than white offending.

The authoritarian father-figure is seen by probation officers as an important influence on crime and occurs in numerous forms.

Such a tendency was found in the content analysis described in the West Midlands in 1987, where the presentation of black people as suffering from weak family units was also clearly evident. As the authors of this study argue, it is questionable whether social histories presented in this manner have relevance to the offence recommendation or justify inclusion in the report.

By referring to earlier records, probation officers can separate themselves to some extent from more unqualified individualised descriptions of personality, as the following extract from a social-enquiry report on a young black offender charged with theft suggests:

> Earlier records indicate an authoritarian and aloof father figure who has become increasingly intolerant towards his family over the years. For years there has been tension at home and I understand that a divorce is likely.

Similarly in another report a probation officer writes:

> Earlier records indicate that X was somewhat spoiled as a child when young. From an early age it was clear that his adoptive father was very punitive and used beating as the usual form of corrective action.

The words 'aloof' and 'authoritarian' in the first report and the description of a punitive father in the second present the black father as a hard, almost inhuman character. One must question how qualified the officers were to use such sweeping terms in relation to the fathers in these cases. For instance, how often was beating used? How does the probation officer know that this was the 'usual' form of correction? Words like authoritarian and aloof are also highly subjective and open to wide interpretation. Such terms need to be carefully qualified or substituted for a form of expression which is more directly related to the alleged offence.

Probation officers in their representation of black offenders in social-enquiry reports appeared to combine conventional explanations in which the black offender is victimised with a less conventional mode of explanation. One probation officer writes of a black offender:

> He has one similar offence but this needs to be seen in the context of the situation, which was basically defending his father and brother, who had been attacked by a rival gang using crow bars.

It would appear that when all else fails X has resorted to violence and has developed a tough image to go with this, which would seem to command the respect of his friends.

In referring to the offender's attack, the probation officer initially emphasises the defensive nature of the offender's reaction. This serves to victimise the subject of the social-enquiry report. Later in the same sentence, the probation officer mentions the fact that this violent posturing commands the respect of his friends. The first part of the quotation presents the subject in terms of oppression, while the second section demonstrates how the violent action has contributed towards the creation of a tough image, which is instrumental in the creation of a positive peer-group identity. It emerged in conversation with the officer that racism contextualised the offence, yet the black offender is portrayed as using violence to create a macho image.

The tendency for probation officers to deflect attention from the impact of racism was noted in the previous chapter, when the work of other researchers was discussed. In the West Midlands study of 1987, after the mention of racial taunts in a social-enquiry report, the probation officer noted the offender's propensity to 'perceive himself as a victim of circumstance'. The independent assessor made a further comment that could equally be applied to the findings of this research:

No attempt was made to present racism as a continuing and ever present feature of the lives of black people, nor any condemnation of the racist incident which resulted in the offence. Racism and its effects are reduced to an over reaction on the part of the client.

(West Midlands 1987: 6)

Pinder would not take this approach, since he describes the probation officers in his sample as attempting to present the logic of black offending in an authentic manner, having regard for the relative emphasis placed upon contributory factors by the offender.

THE PRESENTATION OF THE BLACK FAMILY

Four probation officers from the sample presented the black family in what can only be described as a form which appeared to correspond to populist stereotypical representations of black personality. In all these cases, a distinction was made between the first generation law–abiding parent and the recalcitrant second generation. In describing an offender's mother, an officer made the following observation during an interview:

> Well his mother . . . it's the way she talks, it's the sort of thing you hear parodies of on TV. She's very religious, talks about the preacher, says that she has never been in trouble, and has never caused trouble . . . (pause) . . . they can't understand why their son is like he is. They really are like the stereotypical, conforming, law abiding West Indians who believe in the values of British society. They have hung on and never been a burden to anyone.

What is particularly interesting is the use of the word parody, which could suggest a number of possibilities. The first produces the conclusion that the person mentioned in the quotation can be ascribed to the category of the stereotypical black woman, while second, the officer appears to recognise the parody or misrepresentation. However, he utilises this representation of reality as a mode of understanding. Since this probation officer had no direct experience of interacting with black people beyond his 'professional' capacity, he relies on a representation of the black person derived from the media.

This oversimplified use of the word stereotype appears to suggest that black people with whom the officer comes into contact could possibly conform to such images. Thus the first generation is seen as being duped, conforming to British values which 'probably never existed'. If this is the case, it would seem to follow that second generation black people are acting in a rational manner when they contravene the law. This theme was developed with a different emphasis by another officer who related the logic of second generation black resistance in a white society to his job as a white probation officer. He said in interview:

> I don't know whether it's my phrase or not, but the feeling that black people are the stormtroopers of the working class is a phrase that I have in mind quite a lot.
> DD: What do you understand by that term?
> PO: It's something about a refusal to be actually told your place and stick to it.

Such an explicit statement expressed in societal terms supporting black people was not seen elsewhere in the research. Despite the frequent use of racial stereotypes, which occurred on some 15 occasions if data from all the sources are considered, a form of explanation appears to emerge in descriptions of black families which is highly individualised and does not conform to any identifiable form of conventional explanation. This was particularly evident in relation to descriptions of black religion. It is important to note that the question of religion was not mentioned in any of the material examined on white offenders. The following explanation of religion was given during an interview:

> Mrs X is a fundamentalist, very into her religion which is off putting for X, I feel a bit alienated. I feel uneasy with this. She has asked about getting into the prison to set up groups in there. I was there the other morning and I noticed she had a certificate for evangelical endeavour.
> DD. Who appears to have responsibility for X (the defendant)?
> PO. She has the main responsibility for X.
> DD. What is father's position in the family?
> PO. He is authoritarian, a disciplinarian. He is wheeled in to beat X if he is bad.

A similar sense of alienation is not present in the more official impression created of the same offender in the social-enquiry report:

> Home is a well kept council flat, on a local housing estate. X's parents both work, and appear to manage their finances well. Neither parent has been before the courts, and indeed Mrs X despairs that her son 'won't take any telling from us'. Despite their attempts to give him advice, it is perhaps notable that the offences for which X was convicted all occurred at a time when he was living away from the family home.

While the report represents the offender's parents as responsible adults, the interview illustrates the probation officer's alienation. When the fundamentalism of Mrs X is described as 'off putting for X' this statement is followed by the exclamation: 'I feel a bit alienated'. No evidence was presented to suggest that the offender found his mother's fundamentalism alienating. The probation officer's visits were uncomfortable occasions during which the very topic identified as being a problem for the offender – his mother's religion – is avoided. If religion is defined as a problem for the offender, it seems difficult to account for its avoidance.

The findings of this research suggest that accounts of black families contained ambiguities not present in descriptions of white family forms. This was particularly evident with regard to the notion of the 'dislocated' black family, which was most frequently portrayed in pathological terms. White probation officers appeared to compare black parenting to white imaginary standards of care. It was in describing a black family in a part b record that pathology was linked explicitly to black parenting.

> Just recently X has been the main source of anxiety, truanting from school. I have threatened to ban him from the games room if this goes on, my most potent sanction. I have seen the parents once more and had quite a long chat with dad, but little success in persuading them to take a softer line with the boys – mum wondered if she could have X put away in a home for not going to school! West Indian parents seem to be the main cause of delinquency.

Significantly, this entry was brought to the attention of the researcher by a probation officer who, having taken over super-vision of this family, had been alarmed at what he had found in the record.

THE PERCEIVED INFLUENCE OF THE FAMILY ON WHITE OFFENDING

In describing the family backgrounds of white offenders, proba-tion officers appeared to adopt a more detailed and sympathetic approach, which frequently related to a history of 'bad relationships' within the white offender's family. In a case of assault, the defendant was seen as offending because of an inability to accept the rejection of personal relationships within the family. The following extract from a social-enquiry report characterises such a linkage:

> From the above account, the conclusion may follow that X's offending behaviour originates in his family and social circum-stances where offending at his present age seems endemic. These influences have been heavily reinforced by personal factors, notably deep feelings of inadequacy, and by the punishments that his offending has attracted.

Here offending is conceptualised in terms of the offender being a victim of numerous circumstances including endemic crime. In this case reference is made to personal weakness within the offender, when the inability to cope with personal relationships is mentioned. Another reference is made to the offender's deep feelings of inadequacy. This white offender, like a number of previous black offenders mentioned, is a victim who is presented with an emotive dimension: the weak personality.

This point is important when considered in relation to Pinder's findings. He reported a tendency for probation officers to describe white 'problem' families in terms of a breakdown in personal inter-relationships, while black families appear to be dislocated and aberrant. In other accounts of white offenders, probation officers appeared to focus on descriptions of various forms of loss. This was particularly evident in relation to the white family and was more distinctively represented in accounts given of white than black offenders. The following extract from a social-enquiry report exemplifies the approach:

> X is the youngest of four children. Her parents divorced in 1975, after a long period of marital disharmony. Her father was remarried and she has occasional contact with him. Following this, the mother qualified as an occupational therapist, and is now working in that profession. The defendant has regular contact with her mother but has as yet been unable to tell her of the current probation order, and the fresh offence. Part of my supervision with her has concentrated on helping her to come to terms with residual ambivalent feelings towards her mother, by whom she has felt rejected over the years. It seems that her mother has struggled to be a single parent, as well as develop her own career.

The report goes on to describe the way in which her mother's new relationship has led to the impression being gained by the offender that she has been pushed out and has been led towards a 'deep-rooted insecurity'. She then turned to alcohol as an emotional crutch, which led to offending. Such a line of argument can be expressed in the following way.

THE 'ANTI-AUTHORITARIAN' OFFENDER

References in social-enquiry reports to black anti-authoritarianism came in numerous forms. The term anti-authority refers to the implication that the offender's criminal behaviour can in some respects be related to a tendency to rebel and reject all forms of authority within society. Such an explanation is exemplified in the description contained within a social-enquiry report on a black offender:

> X's pattern of offending in his teenage years seemed consistent with the rebellious and angry behaviour which he demonstrated as a child.

The only redeemable observation made by the officer was that:

> He blames no-one but himself and takes responsibility for what he has done, good or bad.

When the anti-authoritarian offender was conceptualised in these

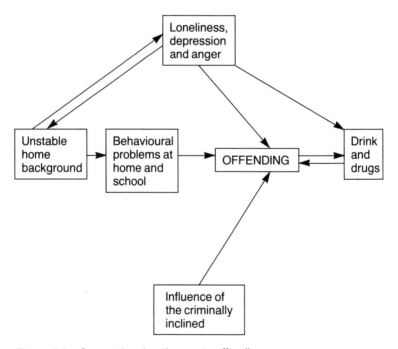

Figure 2.2   Conventional pathways to offending

terms, the notion was frequently contained within a series of negative descriptions creating the impression that social-work intervention is difficult if not impossible. A black female offender despite 'bags of input' in an interview was described as having an authority problem which was:

> Still a threat . . . she seems to resent anyone putting pressure on her to do anything.

The last quotation encapsulates the 'authority problem', which was used to denote what the probation officer perceived to be a clearly defined social phenomenon as distinct from a form of personality or character disorder. The 'authority problem' was seen as stemming from an unexplained resentment and apathy which had a limiting effect on the viability of effective social-work intervention. The theme of resentment was taken up again in a report in which a black youth was charged with actual bodily harm. Meetings between the probation officer and offender were described in the report as being strained and confrontational, with the defendant questioning what probation had to offer him. This is followed by mention of the offender's:

> Resentment at being convicted for an offence where he believed the victim asked for what he got.

The obvious omission from this report was the essential information relating to the background to the offence. It emerged in the interview, as in a previous example, that this offender had been subjected to racial taunts which constituted a vital piece of information. The probation officer chose not to include this information in the report.

All references to anti-authoritarianism were critical, suggesting that the offender's attitude towards criminal activity was beyond the realms of normal understanding. Thus the rejection of authority was seen as an individual defect: no attempt was made to understand the possible causes of such feelings when they were genuinely expressed. One officer dissented from this view and applauded what he saw as the black offender's resistance to oppressive state activity.

White offenders were not described in terms of being anti-authoritarian but occasionally 'reckless' or 'impulsive'. This effectively separated white offenders from the authority problem as described in relation to black offenders.

RACISM AS AN EXPLANATION FOR OFFENDING

It was notable that racism was explicitly used on only three occasions to explain offending in social-enquiry reports. One of these examples has previously been mentioned in the section on the family. References to racism were fairly brief, as the following extract from one of the other reports indicates:

> The defendant's first offence was for stealing a bicycle while staying with his father. There followed two assaults, which it is alleged were a response to racial abuse.

Here an open-ended statement clearly leaves room for doubt as to whether racism was directly connected with the offence. The statement emphasises the fact that racism is alleged by the defendant.

Probation officers appeared reluctant to cite racism as an explanation for offending in an official document; when it was brought to the attention of the court it was usually done so in a brief and somewhat cryptic manner. The possible reasons for this are complex and will be discussed in the next chapter. Probation officers spoke of racism in a more detailed manner during interviews. In the following interview, the explicitness with which racism was discussed can be demonstrated:

> DD: How would you account for X being in trouble with the law?
>
> PO: The reason that he was on probation was about racism, his anger welled up about the fact that people were taunting him, so that in that sense racism can be seen as directly connected with his offending.
>
> DD: Who was taunting him?
>
> PO: Some white students, I think they were poly students.

In the social-enquiry report, however, no mention is made of this element contributing to the offending behaviour. In another interview, in reply to the question as to whether race had been raised as an issue in conversations with the offender, the probation officer replied:

> He feels victimised by the police, he feels that the fact that he is black means that he is picked up on more occasions. The service itself is a part of this authoritarianism, yes, he has very strong feelings about race.

Here it is significant that the officer seems to be tenuously connecting police victimisation and the probation service in his explanation. The offender is presented as combining a critique of both agencies, one coercive, the other consensual. Together they constitute a cocktail of 'authoritarianism' which is then linked back to race. Despite the sensitive interpretation of the offender's perception in structural terms, racism was not mentioned in the social-enquiry report as a possible explanation for offending.

In another interview the following account was given of the way in which the officer had addressed the question of racism in an interview:

> We've addressed the issue of racial harassment, and it has been very difficult to clarify, but I felt that acknowledging his blackness and linking it to his offending behaviour was important for him.

In this case no mention was made regarding the importance of racism to the offender in the social-enquiry report, despite the fact that in the records the question is raised on at least four occasions by the offender as a causal factor which he related to his criminal activities.

Racism was mentioned five times in interviews, but only three times in part c records and was absent in part b records. When racism was raised in records it was given more detailed attention than in social-enquiry reports. In the part c records of a young black offender, the following account of offending behaviour was found:

> He had been charged with theft, which apparently consisted of him carrying a cassette out of an electrical hi-fi store, and waving it about outside at the manager. Apparently the defendant did this in order to prove that the manager was a racist.

Such explicit accounts of an offender's own feelings about racism were rarely found in the research material. An examination of a file on this offender failed to reveal any mention of racism in any other official records or in accounts given to the courts in social-enquiry reports.

The apparent reluctance to explore racism as an explanation for crime could suggest that probation officers feel apprehensive about committing their thoughts about racism to paper. This view would be supported by the lack of reference to racism in social-enquiry reports. The relatively anonymous and informal nature of the interview allowed officers to raise issues related to racism.

IRRESPONSIBILITY

When referring to irresponsibility as possibly influencing offending behaviour, probation officers appeared to be describing a form of action perceived to be entirely irrational and unpredictable, characterised by a lack of any sense of obligation to anyone except themselves. The notion of the irresponsible offender, like that of the authoritarian offender, occurred frequently in reports on black clients, but was absent from reports on white clients. During interviews, one probation officer mentioned irresponsibility as a factor leading towards offending in the case of a white offender.

Irresponsibility was not mentioned as an explanatory factor during interviews with respect to black offenders, although it was mentioned in one interview in relation to a white offender. In social-enquiry reports, irresponsibility was not used in an entirely negative way when attempting to explain black offending, as the following extract from a social-enquiry report on a black offender indicates:

Mr X accepts that he has behaved irresponsibly, the other matters put before the court similarly reflect this.

The probation officer goes on in the report to argue that the realisation of this irresponsibility can be used to appeal to the mercy of the court. She continues:

However, Mr X's recent offending behaviour does not fall into the same category as his previous offending history. He now recognizes that it is as deeply unacceptable, and anti-social, and that consequences for offending are as great.

Thus the realisation of irresponsibility leads to a contrite attitude, which enables the court to use what Walker and Beaumont refer to as 'mercy and discretion' (Walker and Beaumont, 1981).

In another social-enquiry report on a black offender the probation officer links the lack of responsibility to a lack of intelligence, as perceived in terms of intelligence quotient. The officer writes:

Some factors which the court may wish to take into consideration in reaching this decision (*i.e. the decision not to continue probation*)[1] is the defendant's home background, low I.Q., and possibly diminished sense of responsibility. To assist in this a psychiatric report may be useful in this case.

This report has a different tone. The irresponsibility has a pathological label attached to it, being followed, as it is, by the suggestion that the defendant could be helped by a psychiatrist.

BEING LED INTO CRIME BY PEER GROUPS AND PEER-GROUP PRESSURE

In social-enquiry reports, 12 probation officers cited the influence of peer-group pressure as being a significant factor in explaining offending behaviour. It occurred with twice the frequency in reports on white offenders than it did on black offenders. In the case of white offenders this link was made quite explicit as the following extract from a social-enquiry report on a young white offender demonstrates:

> When short of money the defendant appears to have found himself influenced into crime by his co-accused, who was, as far as I know, the instigator of these offences.

This was the more usual manner in which offenders were conceptualised as being led into crime. No social-enquiry report was found in which the subject was leading others into crime. In another social-enquiry report on a young white offender the link between the influence of peers and offending is also made quite explicit:

> The original offences, however, took place in the company of X, a young man who lived near the defendant, and who is very well known for his persistent thieving. This influence was very bad, and although the defendant is no longer acquainted with X, it seems that stealing from shops is persisting with him.

This reference serves to diminish the responsibility that the offender has for the offence, while still allowing the probation officer leeway to acknowledge the seriousness of the offence. It is clearly an effective device in court, used by probation officers when trying to argue for a non–custodial sentence. This theme is not developed in other forms of data on white offenders. In describing the influence of a peer group on a black offender, the social-enquiry report reads as follows:

> Mr X does not have a serious history of offending. The trouble he has been in reflects the changes in his life since leaving the security and supervision of the children's home, and in particular that since his move to X, he has mixed in with quite a delinquent group of young men. Given his employment prospects the chances of further trouble must be reasonably high.

Generally, there was no appreciable qualitative difference in the way in which this explanation of offending was presented in reports on black or white offenders. It was the frequency with which this form of explanation occurred, clearly favouring white offenders, which was significant.

DEPRESSION

The notion of depression was constructed from the language of medicine. Reactive depression was regarded as resulting from a specific traumatic event such as a major bereavement. Thus by definition the condition tended to be thought of in temporary terms, since the person suffering from such a form of depression could recover with help and with the passing of time. The causes of endogenous depression were not always apparent and were frequently seen to be indicative of a more far-reaching fundamental psychiatric problem, possibly of a permanent nature. From an examination of the research material it appeared that probation officers were more likely to present the former form of depression as contributing to offending behaviour. In one case a white offender was seen to be suffering from 'acute' depression which seemed to indicate a 'disease' characterised by 'a sudden onset, but of short duration'.

In social-enquiry reports written on white offenders, depression was used as an explanation of offending on four occasions, but it only appeared once in a social-enquiry report written on a black offender. A further dimension is added to this in that when depression was used it tended to be seen in relation to white women. An example of the way in which depression was used as an explanation of offending in social-enquiry reports can be seen in a report written on X, a 20-year-old white woman offender:

> The defendant acknowledges that when she keeps appointments with me she finds our discussions helpful and supportive, she has some insight into her deep-rooted insecurity, and her resultant patterns of behaviour that still cause her problems from time to time, particularly with regard to relationships. I believe the offences last year which led to this order were committed during a period of depression, while struggling to cope with independence and loneliness. It would also seem that her money management was bad because she was spending too much on alcohol as an emotional crutch.

This social-enquiry report is a variant on the line of argument frequently used in the case of white offenders to explain behaviour. The use of depression in this 'medical' manner explains the offence in terms of a disease – depression, which renders the sufferer unable to take full responsibility for her actions. Since depression is temporary and essentially reactive, the hope of recovery makes the possibility of successful probation intervention a viable proposition for the court to consider. Here depression is related to drinking. The need for drink leads to undue expenditure on alcohol, which then creates a further need for offending behaviour in order to pay for more drink. It has already been noted that such cyclical forms of argument were not as evident in explanations of black offending.

In the only case in which depression was used to explain black offending the following presentation was made to the court:

> The defendant tells me that there were his first offences and adds that he has never received so much as a caution. On this occasion he had been riding his pedal-cycle down the shopping centre listening to music through head-phones, something that he says he does frequently when he is feeling depressed. He threw a drain grid through a shop window on each occasion and stole watches and items of clothing from the displays. I gather that some of these goods were recovered. The defendant adds that they were items he neither wanted nor needed, and can offer no explanation for what he says are spontaneous acts of folly.

Here the probation officer presents the offending behaviour in such a way as to lead the reader towards the view of the offender as an incorrigible youth who acts irrationally, stealing items that he does not want or need. The worst effects of the potentially damaging image of the recalcitrant youth riding his bicycle listening to headphones, and mindlessly throwing a drain grid through a shop front, is ameliorated to a large extent by the use of the word 'depressed' which is perhaps the only possible way in which the probation officer could make such an act understandable to the courts. The report continues:

> Previous reports have linked the defendant's offending to the depressing, and disturbing home situation, and certainly his mother's over-protectiveness, and his father's tendency to over-react and punish him have not helped. However, I feel that the defendant is now beginning to realise that he has to accept responsibility for the actions himself, and I see his current difficulty as situational, as well as indicative of wider social problems. The first offence occurred when the defendant met a friend and was persuaded to accept a car lift, knowing it to be stolen. He now sees that it was foolish to do so, but thought it difficult to back down. Certainly this sort of car offence is not in keeping with the defendant's previous pattern of offending. The other offences are for shop lifting clothes, and I believe are directly related to him losing his job.

Here a rather more brusque account of the black offender's depression is given and, unlike the white offender's depression, does not appear to have been accepted by the officer. It is also significant to note the apparent rejection of black family stereotypical structures which dominated other explanations of crime. The punitive father and overprotective mother are here replaced by a call for realism on the part of the offender to accept the consequences of his actions.

'RELATIONSHIP PROBLEMS' AS AN EXPLANATION FOR OFFENDING BEHAVIOUR

It is necessary at the outset to clarify what is being referred to by the use of the words 'relationship problems'. Reference is being made to problems arising within sexual partnerships. Relationships in the research material were heterosexual in nature. Only one reference was made to homosexuality, where one white offender's daughter had proclaimed her lesbian tendencies which had 'contributed to the offender's sense of isolation'. Probation officers tended to utilise explanations of offending based on relationship problems, most noticeably in part c records. This practice was followed in relation to only one black offender. In this case the offence in the part c records is explained in terms of a violent relationship:

> He talks in the interviews about fights and scuffles over a period of time, which on one occasion resulted in him being cut on the shoulder with a bread knife, he showed me the scar. He also described another occasion in which he alleged that he found her in bed with his father. X clearly puts a great deal into trying to understand and work out this relationship.

Such an emotionally charged account was quite rare in the records and indicates that within his own terms, the probation officer was genuinely attempting to grapple with the emotional state of the offender. A similar approach can be seen in relation to the descriptions of difficulties experienced by white couples.

THE DIMENSION OF GENDER IN EXPLAINING OFFENDING BEHAVIOUR

In two instances offending was related to issues peculiar to gender. In the first case in which a black woman was caught shop-lifting in a supermarket, the following explanation was given:

> X was upset, she had been caught shop-lifting at Y on Friday. She was shopping with her daughter, and at the till put some goods straight into a carrier bag which had been given to her at the till. She said she did not realise what she had done until she was stopped, and outside the store, she offered to pay for the goods, but was refused by the store detective. X says she was feeling unwell, and had got confused, she had period pains and migraine, and the baby was making a fuss. She felt sick and shocked when she was stopped and arrested. At the police station she tried to explain the circumstances, but she tells me that the police were threatening to keep her for a long time, and she was worried about the baby, so she made a statement admitting shop-lifting to get home to her daughter. X is afraid that this matter will come before the court again since she knows she might get a custodial sentence.

Here the probation officer creates the image of a woman overburdened with the responsibilities of child-rearing. The reference to migraine and period pains adds a powerful force to this image, having an arguable effect. On the one hand it can be seen as forming a basis for mitigation. On the other hand such wording can be seen as presenting women in the words of Smart as:

> At the mercy of their anatomy and emotions. Most studies of female offenders refer to women in terms of their biological impulses and hormonal imbalance or in terms of their domesticity, maternal instinct and passivity.
>
> (Smart 1976: 71)

As Worral incisively points out:

> If 'feminine conditions' are recognised only in mitigation and not in defence then their recognition assists the management of female law breakers without conceding authority (or, indeed authenticity) to the women's own accounts.
>
> (Worral 1990: 95)

Such tendencies are reflected in a part b record relating to a black woman offender who is described as having a tendency:

> To shut reality out and live in a nice fantasy world of pretty things, and shelve problems. However, she is beginning for the first time to open out problems that have harboured for years, and she is likely to unearth the roots of her offending behaviour.

In the social-enquiry report and in previous records, reference had been made to the hardships which had been suffered by this offender, yet it was still possible for her to live in a 'nice fantasy world of pretty things in order to shelve problems'. This apparent irrationality will be remedied by the process of 'opening out', which although not defined as an operational concept, would enable her to unearth the roots of problems which underlie her offending behaviour. Such spurious logic, based on often ambiguous and contradictory evidence, raises a number of important problems.

The white woman offender is frequently presented to the courts by the probation officer in terms of being neurotic or irrational, these being the 'true' characteristics of women (Smart 1976). This may well be related to the finding from this research, that the notion of the depressed woman was most frequently attributed to the white woman. Black women are mythically presented as being in some way unpredictable and irrational, while also suffering the effects of institutionalised racism. Probation officers in this research were either unable or unwilling to convey a sense of the structured subordination of black women in their explanations of offending behaviour. Instead a safe, defensive posture was taken by officers which enabled the difficulties faced by women to be contextualised within biological cycles, feminine 'silliness' and random misfortune. The views of the women themselves remained concealed and untapped within the complex language of professional conventionality.

PROVOCATION

Provocation was perceived by probation officers as influencing crime, most notably in social-enquiry reports on black offenders. Although frequently linked with racism, this category of explanation should be regarded as being distinctive for two principal reasons. First, it occurred in one case involving a white offender. Second, it was occasionally used to deflect from racist taunts reported to white probation officers by black offenders. The use of the term provocation serves to remove the reality of racism and its possible link to the commission of a violent act.

In a social-enquiry report in which the provocation of a white offender was emphasised, as was the case with black offenders, it was attributed to peer-group pressure. After a drunken evening in a public house, one white defendant was provoked by a rival white gang. The subject of the report was:

Constantly mocked and spurred on by his own friends to become violent.

There were some important common features frequently presented by probation officers, as constituting provocation for black and white offenders. First, the incidents occurred in public places. Second, there would appear to have been considerable group pressure exerted on offenders immediately before the offence was committed. Third, the probation officer is presenting the provocation as an influence directly affecting the commission of crime: thus without provocation the offence would not have occurred. This has the effect of providing an explanation which is external to the offender. Thus while acknowledging that the violent act itself appears to emanate from the individual, the provoking act diminishes the responsibility that the defendant can take, since the provocation was 'unreasonable'. This enables the probation officer to argue further that the isolated piece of behaviour does not reflect the 'true' nature of the offender. The offending act thus becomes 'unusual' or 'out of character' and can be used in social-enquiry reports to justify a lighter non-custodial sentence.

Although this tendency was evident in material on black and white offenders, racism was frequently an added dimension to the provocation suffered by some black offenders. Despite the central part which racism clearly played in some of these incidents, it was rarely mentioned and never condemned.

This can be seen when the imitation of a black youth's walk was seen by the probation officer as sparking off an attack. This is mentioned in the social-enquiry report as follows:

He tells me that he was initially provoked by the victim of the attack imitating his walk, and that subsequently a heated argument developed.

It also becomes clear in the social-enquiry report that the subject 'struck the victim first'. The officer then goes on to express surprise that the defendant should have acted in this way, commenting that:

I was surprised to learn that X was involved in a violent incident, because there was no indication that he is or has been inclined towards violent behaviour.

During the interview in which the report was being discussed, the probation officer emphasised that this offender was much preoccupied with his 'blackness', and that the incident had been sparked off by a combination of racist abuse and the imitation of the defendant's walk. There is no reference to this in the social-enquiry report, however, although it seems highly probable that the incident which sparked off the attack could more properly be regarded as being associated with racism.

This failure on the part of probation officers to emphasise and condemn some of the worst excesses of racism was also found in previous work already mentioned (Whitehouse 1983; West Midlands study 1987). This may well reflect a reluctance on the part of probation officers to forestall anticipated adverse magisterial or judicial reaction to the condemnation of racism in reports.

PRAGMATIC OFFENDING

Although the probation officers rarely used this term directly in social-enquiry reports, the meaning was made clear in an interview with a probation officer. In discussing a young black offender charged with shop-lifting the probation officer commented:

> X needed the cassette player, so he just took it . . . (pause) . . . it was as simple as that. He walked into a shop, grabbed the player and ran . . . purely pragmatic.

In using the words 'needed' and not 'wanted' it may be possible to argue that the officer was showing some degree of understanding of the position in which the offender found himself. This perceived influence on offending occurred with most regularity in social-enquiry reports on black offenders and was used exclusively in relation to crimes of property, as distinct from crimes connected with the person.

Pragmatic offending was not always expressed in as straight-forward a way as the above example would suggest. In a social-enquiry report on a black offender charged with theft, the following account is given. After losing his job:

> He was used to earning approximately £Y per week, and used to spend most of this on clothes. After being dismissed he received no supplementary benefit and has therefore gone from being reasonably affluent to penniless in a few weeks. He reverted to his old habits and resorted to shoplifting to get things he wanted. He understands that this is no excuse, but it is his explanation of why he reoffended.

This explanation is a more difficult one to present in a social-enquiry report, since it implies that the offender wanted something that he could not obtain legally. Faced with this situation, he simply broke the law to achieve his aims. The condemnatory effect of this is even more forceful since the offending was mentioned in the context of dismissal from employment. The impact of this is ameliorated somewhat since the offender appears to realise that there 'is no excuse' which suggests a degree of contrition, giving the court the opportunity to use their mercy and discretion. This would seem to be the desired result from the probation officer's perspective since he concluded the report by recommending a probation order.

The presentation of pragmatic white offending, although less prevalent, was seen by probation officers in similar terms. In a social-enquiry report written on a young white offender in connection with a charge of shop-lifting, the writer comments:

> X tells me that he needed the items and walked out of the shop with them in his hand without thinking.

Here the goods involved were parts for a motorcycle and cannot be regarded as essential. The subject of the report was currently unemployed but was described in the interview as: 'Having a fetish about his motorbike'. There is a qualitative difference in this account when compared with similar explanations of black offending: the white offender according to his own account was not in real control of his senses when the offence occurred because of fetishism. The act was committed without thinking, which effectively separates the offender from the criminal act. The implication here is that had he been thinking, the offence would not have occurred. This is a similar line of argument to that found in the presentation of provocation, depression, the use of alcohol and most of the major categories of explanation which have been identified, with the obvious exclusion of racism.

There are two forms of pragmatic offending which can be described in the following terms. Rational pragmatic offending is presented as being understandable to the courts if the items stolen are essential and the intention of the theft is not frivolous. Irrational pragmatic offending can be used by probation officers to account for the theft of non-essential luxury goods which provide immediate gratification of wants and not needs. A distinction is being made here in terms of what can broadly be viewed as deserving and undeserving crime. Both forms of explanation were present in the material examined on white and black offenders.

LIFESTYLE

This complex and vague notion appeared in part b records kept on three black offenders, two of whom were women. In one other part b record on a black offender the combination of a high lifestyle and low income was used to account for criminal activity. Attempts were made in the second interview to clarify the notion without much success. It seemed that different officers had different understandings of the term. One officer described lifestyle as being:

> The way in which offenders organise their daily lives, whether they get up early, dress soberly, and formally or just look a mess . . . things like that.

Another probation officer related lifestyle to culture, describing it as being:

> The way in which certain values deriving from culture affect peoples' lives.

In the atmosphere of vagueness it was difficult to reach any understanding on how probation officers saw this concept as contributing to offending.

In one part b record kept on a young black woman, the probation officer noted:

> She says that she won't take the risk of shoplifting again, it's a mug's game, but will handle and receive. Everybody around X is offending. She likes the excitement and lifestyle of it all, it's all she knows.

The patronising and possibly racist tone contained in the words 'it's all she knows' again reveals the extent to which black women are subjected to multiple oppression within the criminal justice system, some of which lacks subtlety and sophistication. The suggestion that she 'likes the excitement' appeared on examination of all the available evidence in probation records to be unsubstantiated.

ANGER

Previous discussion has considered the question of anger in sections on provocation, racism, the family, alcohol and relationships. Anger was presented as a single causal factor in offending behaviour most noticeably in social-enquiry reports on black offenders. In one such report the court was told by the probation officer that:

X's pattern of offending is consistent with angry behaviour as a child.

Anger presented to the court in this way would appear to have negative connotations. The passage suggests a consistency in behaviour which has been present in the individual for the greater part of his life, which would seem to lead to an obvious pessimistic conclusion that nothing can be done for the individual non-custodially. Anger of this type for probation officers cannot be compared to drunkenness or psychiatric illness. It is a feature of individual behaviour which could be curbed with self-control. It appears to follow from this that angry people are less likely to respond to probation. Anger appears to many probation officers to emanate not from situations or from the wider society in which the offender lives, but incubates within the offender's mind manifesting itself in 'Flashpoints of anger which directly relate to offending'. The angry offender could show another side to his personality, in one case transforming himself into a 'gentle giant'.

ACTING OUT BEING A CRIMINAL

This unusual form of explanation occurred in three part c records kept on black offenders. It did not appear in more formal documents like social-enquiry reports, possibly because it was vague and considered by probation officers to be unacceptable as an 'official' explanation of crime. The following extract from a c follower entry on a black male gives an impression of the qualitative nature of this form of explanation:

X is a real showman, when he is being the mature grown up X he shows off in quite amusing ways. When he is being the juvenile immature X he plays to the gang, acting out being the smooth guy. Part of this involves his being the sophisticated criminal. This isn't so funny. Thus in a peer group in which offending is the norm X plays to the audience and in order to gain esteem he offends. This is part of the process of being 'smooth' and 'streetwise', thus defending a strong position within the peer group structure.

In all accounts given of such offending the idea of acting out being a criminal was presented in slightly theatrical terms and linked to peer groups. Perhaps this was the most imaginative of all the explanatory criteria employed by probation officers which seems to have little relation to substantive evidence of any kind. We shall return later to the process of deconstructing constructions of probation reality.

SOME GENERAL COMPARISONS BETWEEN EXPLANATIONS OF OFFENDING FOR BLACK AND WHITE OFFENDING

Having given detailed consideration to particular differences that emerged from all sources of research material it is necessary to make some more generalised comments relating to the differential perceptions of influences on offending, as expressed by probation officers. Although there were variations in explanations provided in social-enquiry reports on white offenders, there was an important unifying strand: the explanations being offered strongly suggested to the court that there were factors out of the offender's control which could potentially create a situation in which the offender was vulnerable to offending behaviour. Such scenarios were largely brought about by the random build-up of external factors. There was also a considerable amount of congruity between explanations offered in social-enquiry reports and interviews, although there were exceptions to this. Explanations for offending in records also bore a striking resemblance to each other in documents relating to white offenders, concentrating on what has been referred to as conventional forms of explanation.

The white offender was frequently presented as a victim of cruel circumstance. This minimised the amount of blame that could be attributed to the individual. Such explanations often constituted a plea for 'one last chance' and in one case the 'mercy of the court'. Although some explanations for offending offered in social-enquiry reports written on black offenders also tended to concentrate on external factors and circumstances acting upon the offender, there were many accounts in which black offenders were presented in a way which was qualitatively different from the explanations associated with white offenders. When discussing black offenders, probation officers tended to combine familiar conventional accounts of offending with differing forms of explanation, which, as has been seen in the section on the family, frequently resorted to the use of stereotype and myth. Underlying all this was a clear reluctance to associate racism with criminal activity. When racism was connected with offending, its effects were minimised.

In some cases the explanations for black offending were even more problematic. Use of the term 'almost instinctive criminality' creates the impression that the black offender possessed an innate propensity for criminal behaviour which was performed without conscious intention. When in the second interview the probation officer was asked why the word 'instinctive' had been used in relation to black offending, he immediately recognised that it could have racist connotations and added:

> The problem is, I do not know whether I would have used the word in relation to a white client.

This response would appear to suggest that the officer acknowledged the existence of racism and the possible racist connotation of terms used in the report. What was apparently unclear to the officer concerned was why such an understanding had not been utilised in practice. In this example it was not just the case that the officer appeared to minimise or ignore racism, but that he voluntarily introduced a concept which was clearly understood after the event as having racist overtones.

This is an important point, since in some of the earlier literature there is the suggestion that the differential treatment of black offenders by white probation officers was attributable to the unquestioning white Eurocentrism of probation officers (e.g. Whitehouse 1983). What appears to emerge is a separation of consciousness between the 'theoretical' world of anti-racist training on social-work courses and the pragmatic task of writing a social-enquiry report in the 'real' world of the criminal justice system. Such a tendency replicates the way in which anti-racist training is often presented to social-work students as a one- or two-day exercise, an activity which is in some way hybrid and separate from everyday social-work activity. The anti-racist 'workshop' is frequently taught by black consultants who are 'called in' to provide the anti-racist 'input'. White social-work tutors are thus separated from this form of 'specialism', and concern themselves with the reality of other substantive areas of social-work theory and practice. In many cases little effort is made to utilise what students have learned on the anti-racist day, even though students have been profoundly affected by the experience. It is not surprising that anti-racist practice is not structured into social-work activity but becomes marginal to everyday social-work tasks.

In another social-enquiry report regarding a charge of burglary,

the defendant's work record is seen as being 'abysmal' and he is seen
as having a low IQ which could possibly lead to a diminished sense
of responsibility. Such a presentation links black offending to a low
IQ, an association that has little meaning.

It was argued earlier that explanations given of white offending
in social-enquiry reports were similar to those given in the unstructured interviews and records kept by probation officers. The same
point cannot be made in relation to many of the explanations given
of black offending. In the following case the client's own definition
of the situation was given quite forcefully during the interview.
Here we see that the police 'picked on' the offender, which seems
to have been a significant contributing factor in explaining his
offending behaviour:

> DD: How do you account for the position in which X finds
>   himself?
> PO: He would say that the police pick on him. He has recently
>   been picked up by the police, and he attributes many of
>   his problems to police attitudes. I think that he has a point
>   here. I generally agree with him about the police.

In the social-enquiry report, however, there is no mention of the
police. The following account is given of his offending behaviour:

> He has little to say regarding the offences that he appears before
> the court for today. The offences all occurred in March of this
> year, so he has had plenty of time to reflect on his behaviour. He
> admits that he knew it was wrong to take someone else's push
> bike, but needed bits for his own, and knew that his mother could
> not afford to buy them for him. He now very much regrets this
> behaviour and assures me that he will not be tempted in this
> way again.

Here once again the split is evident between the explanation offered
by the officer in the less formal reality of the interview and the
official reality of the social-enquiry report.

In the case of one black offender there were no fewer than four
different explanations given for offending in the four sources of data
that were examined, i.e. the explanation for crime in social-enquiry
reports, interview and records. In the social-enquiry report the
following explanation is given:

> She generally finds that her outgoings exceed her income, and

fails to exercise the rigorous financial restraint required to live within her means. She strives to maintain a child, a household, and herself in a meticulous manner on a limited budget. This situation leaves her vulnerable to offending.

In the part c records, however, we find the following explanation of offending:

> The defendant was shopping and at the till the defendant put some goods straight into a carrier bag which had been given to her at the till, she says she did not realise what she had done until she was stopped outside the store, and offered to pay, but was refused.

In the part b records we see the following explanation:

> The defendant re-offended within five weeks of the probation order commencing, and this places her in a very pressurized position. Shop-lifting is an integral part of her life, which she was introduced to by her step-mother and continues to be concerned with alongside other members of her family. She struggles alone to provide for herself, and her three-year-old daughter.

In interview, however, the probation officer commented:

> She finds herself in a very insecure, and confused position, and frequently has periods in which she is unable to control certain impulses which lead her towards shop-lifting.

A number of different explanations are being given for this example of female crime. In the social-enquiry report, as Worral notes, domestic problems are seen in courts as explaining and possibly excusing female crime (Worral 1990). The assumption that crime is in some way structured into the life of an offender, or is controlled by an inexplicable and mysterious impulse, exemplifies both the power and freedom exercised by probation officers in descriptions of black women. Although by presenting the client's 'weakness' in domestic terms, the probation officer in this case was arguably attempting to present a view of the woman and the offence which he considered to be acceptable to the courts. If we view this explanation with the other less formal explanations we are faced with an absurdly bewildering and inconsistent catalogue of female 'weaknesses'.

PHYSICALITY AND THE BLACK OFFENDER

Although it cannot be said that white probation officers attempted to explain black offending in terms of black physicality, a number of direct references were made to the powerful effect of a black physical presence. Accounts of white physicality were not present in the material. One probation officer commented in interview:

X has a very physical presence . . . he is dominant, strong, and very black.

Another black offender was described in interview as:

Laid back, very good looking, tall, very smart, and a sharp dresser.

Reference was also made to a black offender as being:

Very large, he makes an immense physical impression.

Although the physical presence was not directly related to offending, it occurred in spontaneously in some seven interviews when offending was being discussed.

It should be emphasised that black physicality was not mentioned in social-enquiry reports. In statements of an unofficial nature, probation officers appeared to find a continuity between black identity and a black physical appearance. Black people were being characterised in terms of the perceived power of their physical appearance. In the West Midlands study (1987) such links were made more formally in social-enquiry reports. Here, as was noted in Chapter 1, evidence was found directly linking a 'well-built and strong Afro-Caribbean' with 'getting into trouble with the law'.

Chapter 3

Social-work practice with black and white offenders

In this chapter the nature of probation work with black and white offenders will be comparatively considered. A number of questions have been formulated arising from a concern to understand the possible effect of racism or anti-racism on probation practice. These questions also relate to some of the issues raised in the previous chapter, which sought to explore probation officers' perceptions of offending behaviour. This chapter, then, focuses on the process of probation work with black and white offenders.

It is first necessary to specify what is meant by the process of social work. Although this is an area of great contention, a working model which helps to clarify the notion of process has been recently developed by Preston-Shoot and Williams. They have described a series of steps which they argue constitute an evaluative form of process in social work which is as follows:

1 A description of the situation as precisely as possible.
2 A description of the broad aim of the work with a desired outcome.
3 The identification of feasible objectives.
4 A description of the intervention designed to achieve the desired objective.
5 The identification of indicators which reveal change.
6 A decision as to who will record what and why.
7 Establish the plan for evaluating steps 1–6.
8 Review the results of the intervention prior to either a return to step 1 or termination and subsequent follow-up.

(Preston-Shoot and Williams 1987)[1]

Although no formulation can be free from criticism, the clarity of this model creates a useful guideline for the basis of a planned and systematic process in social work. For the probation officer, the first step in the probation-work process of intervention is the formulation of a recommendation in a social-enquiry report which inevitably constitutes an assessment and a recommendation for court disposal based upon the probation officer's assessment.

This would be followed by a more formal assessment, usually recorded in the part b record, which in this research for white offenders was not dissimilar from the social-enquiry report assessment. The next process would be the carrying out of the intervention based on the assessment. Evidence of the day-to-day progress of this was found in the part c records and from personal accounts given by probation officers during interview. The third process involves the officer in a process of evaluating the intervention in order to understand the effectiveness of the work. Evidence of this was sought in all records and in interviews. Put simply we are attempting to ascertain whether the intervention had the effect desired or anticipated by the probation officer. In addressing the issues that arise from my own research, the following questions have been formulated, which will structure the chapter.

1 Was there any evidence to suggest that probation officers made qualitatively different forms of recommendations in social-enquiry reports when black and white offenders were examined in detail?
   This question is concerned with the complex relationship between the formation of arguments in social-enquiry reports and sentencing decisions.

2 Was there any difference between black and white assessments and proposed practice plans?
   Much of the work of the probation officer is linked to the assessment process which warrants examination since it is a primary social-work task.
   The researcher wished to establish whether probation officers' assessments constituted a basis for social work and whether the assessment did bear any relation to the form of practice undertaken.

3 Was there a comparative difference in the way in which day-to-day work was undertaken with white and black offenders?

Here aspects of probation practice which emerged from the
research will be examined.

4 Did probation officers measure the effectiveness of their work
   with black and white offenders differentially?
   This question was posed in order to draw attention not only to
   the process of intervention but also to the outcome for offenders.
   Outcome in this sense refers to the results of social-work intervention, in other words, the possible benefits and/or disadvantages
   which accrue to the offender as a direct result of contact with the
   probation service.

5 Were black offenders seen by probation officers as posing any
   particular problems which might lead them to be less optimistic
   about the viability of intervention?
   An attempt is being made here to ascertain whether probation
   officers regard black offenders as having characteristics which
   create problems for the probation officers' work.

PROBATION OFFICERS' RECOMMENDATIONS IN
RELATION TO BLACK AND WHITE OFFENDING

One of the most powerful features of the probation officer's job is
the writing of social-enquiry reports. The most important section
of the report is the final recommendation. In this section the relationships between final recommendations and arguments contained
in the body of reports will be examined. In the previous chapter
it was argued that when writing social-enquiry reports probation
officers will catalogue a number of explanations for offending,
which constitute what was referred to as a conventional form
of explanation. The purpose of this is effectively to distance the
offender from the offending behaviour; or, according to Pinder,
to use conventional forms of 'excuse' to account for the behaviour
(Pinder 1984).

Probation officers combine this with a tendency to use such explanations to victimise the offender. Thus reasons are sought to account
for the offending behaviour which will make a recommendation for
non-custodial disposal rational to the sentencer. In other words,
when probation officers make conventional recommendations they
tend to use excusing or victimising terms.

Although these comments can be applied to reports on both black and white offenders to some extent, there emerged a qualitative difference in the way in which the explanations were presented. In cases involving young black offenders, conventional rules of 'professional' argument were modified for a number of possible reasons. The form in which the report is written may be affected by racism on the part of the writer, or the desire to present a black view of social reality which incorporates racism. The central question that emerges is the relationship between the form of explanation for offending and the recommendation made by the probation officer to the court. It is important to recognise that for a probation officer writing social-enquiry reports, the sequencing of arguments and the relation between particular sequencing and recommendations constitute a major part of their social-work practice. This problem will now be explored by examining in detail the accounts given by probation officers in social-enquiry reports.

The following case of shop-lifting involving a young white woman offender will exemplify the 'conventional' relationship between explanations of offending and recommendations. The sequence of explanations in the report can be expressed thematically as follows.

The recommendation for probation reads as follows:

X presents as an anxious frightened young woman, who sees herself as 'a victim of circumstance'. The previous probation order helped her practically to become more assertive, and create some form of control over her own life. Unfortunately she appears to be back to square one. I would therefore suggest to the court that a further probation order be appropriate in this case, especially as X is very isolated at the moment, and needs a confidante to help her make decisions and change her life for the better.

1 She was under considerable stress.
↓
2 She wanted to draw attention to her plight.
↓
3 Her husband was increasingly violent towards her.
↓
4 Non-custodial recommendation by probation officer.
↓
5 Non-custodial disposal by the courts.

Figure 3.1 To show conventional representation of events in relation to shop-lifting

There are a number of observations about this report which help exemplify what has been referred to in this research as conventional practice. The recommendation clearly relates to the forms of explanation which have been provided earlier in the report. The defendant is afraid of a violent husband. This is presented as a circumstance and not a form of individual pathology. The offence is then removed from the essential personality of the individual since she was attempting to draw attention to these circumstances. The report does not enable the reader to learn why it is that the individual expresses her anxiety through crime.

The probation officer then identifies what the offender needs. The offender requires more assertiveness and control over adverse circumstances which dominate her life and lead her towards offending. This link between the need for control over her situation and the role of the probation officer was previously achieved as a result of a probation order, although no evidence is given in the report as to how the previous officer was able to work with the offender. It then becomes possible for the probation officer to present the offence in terms of regression by referring to her as being 'back to square one'. The work previously carried out with this offender did not have a permanent effect since she has again found herself before the courts. Having established and justified the need for probation, a role for the probation officer is expressed in terms of the worker becoming a 'confidante'.

Thus probation can be seen as solving problems for this offender as catalogued in the probation officer's explanations of the offence. The stress, lack of control, regression, violent husband and anxiety can be solved by the probation officer becoming a confidante. It could be argued that such an explanation and recommendation is an ambitious project which places an enormous pressure on one worker, and that the argument leading to the recommendation was somewhat lacking in credibility. What seems to be important, however, is that the report follows an acceptable line of 'conventional' logic, even if some obvious questions are left unanswered. Explanations for offending are related to the recommendation which should contain a solution to the problems faced by the offender. An undue confidence is invested in the one-to-one form of work which is implied by the notion of the confidante. This is acceptable to the courts since it is enshrined within the conditions of the probation order in which the individual officer's role is to 'advise, assist and befriend'.

In another example of conventional report-writing, a picture of a confused background is presented to the court:

With a history of familial disharmony, and a school career which was characterised by truancy despite 'normal intelligence'.

Although this white offender has entered a plea of 'not guilty' the probation officer mounts an elaborate case for probation based on conventional lines. After the defendant has been found guilty he writes:

I am recommending that the court take note of Mr X's desire to change although I am aware of two difficulties with this. His co-defendant in this case has received a custodial sentence for the same offences in which Mr X was involved. Secondly the defendant continues to affirm his innocence. In my opinion this should not be an insuperable obstacle to effective supervision. Should the court agree to a non-custodial sentence there are a number of options. I first considered community service, but I do not feel that this is what the defendant needs. The defendant needs further help and guidance. His desire to stay out of trouble is not assisted by the inconsistencies which he experiences at home. At the same time I have put aside the possibility of placing the defendant in a probation hostel since the pull of home is too strong, and whilst his difficulties have been exacerbated by home factors they are probably best resolved there and not in the hostel. Similarly I have considered the day probation programme, which may place more stress on the defendant than he is able to take at the present time, since he has only just come round to being able to discuss his personal life. He also hopes to register with an industrial training programme, the restart scheme. The day probation programme would prevent his attendance on this course. I would therefore ask the court to consider a non-custodial sentence, and that a conventional probation order should be granted. Such supervision would be in accordance with a specific contract the terms of which I have already discussed with the client.

There are a number of observations to be made about this recommendation. Despite the defendant's continued efforts to 'affirm his innocence' the probation officer feels strongly enough about the case to recommend probation in a forcible manner. The fact that the offender does not acknowlege his guilt is not for this probation officer an 'insuperable obstacle' to probation. Having established the need for a non-custodial sentence, the probation officer then eliminates the various sentencing options. He reaches the conclusion that the offender needs social-work intervention since he has expressed a 'desire to change'. One of the important explanations provided by the probation officer was the home circumstances of the defendant which had exacerbated his difficulties. These problems are made to appear soluble at home by the rejection of the idea of the offender being placed in a hostel.

This further strengthens the case for a non-custodial sentence since the view that the offender's problems can be best solved at home gives the impression that there is something further to be gained by not imposing a custodial sentence. The rejection of the day-probation-programme option gives the opportunity to inform the court that the defendant has recently started to discuss his personal life. The implication here is that he can do this on a one-to-one basis but not in a group, which further promotes the idea of a conventional probation order. The rejection of the day-probation programme as a sentencing option also enables the probation officer to introduce the fact that the offender has applied for a government scheme, which is further proof of his desire to direct himself towards a more industrious lifestyle.

Earlier in the recommendation the probation officer strongly asserted that the defendant 'needed' help and guidance. This theme is referred to at the end of the report when the recommendation is actually made, since the probation officer requests a conventional probation order in which work will be contractually based. The sentencer could gain the impression that this is a viable proposition since the terms of the contract have already been agreed with the defendant.

The accumulative effect of this lengthy recommendation is threefold. First, it makes probation a viable and attractive option for a sentencer. Second, it eliminates other sentencing options. Third, a clear message is given to the sentencer that the defendant is anxious to change. In this recommendation the probation officer has shown what may almost be described as a determination to have the defendant placed on probation. Every attempt has been made to cover all interpretations of the defendant's behaviour: the reader is led to the inevitable conclusion that in this case probation is an appropriate and effective form of disposal.

When recommendations were made for community service in the case of white offenders the tone of the reports tended to be positive, both in relation to the offenders' relationship with the probation service and to the likelihood of community service being a successful and viable sentencing option. This would be expected since in making a 'high tariff' recommendation, sentencers require substantive reasons for following this option. Such a positive image is given in the way in which the following argument for community service is synthesised.

> I supervised the offender previously on parole licence. He was always co-operative and I had no cause to worry about his life in general. His co-operative response has been a feature of his relationship with the probation service over recent years. My overall impression of the defendant is that he has emerged from a troublesome adolescence, and shows every sign of being a responsible adult both in terms of employment and within the home. My observations to date lead me towards a very positive picture. I can confirm his suitability for a community service order.

In this recommendation reference is made to the positive relationship the offender has previously had with probation officers. The reader learns that the offender has emerged from a 'troubled' adolescence and shows signs of rehabilitation, although no evidence is given to support this observation. The previous positive intervention does not appear to have prevented the new offences from taking place. With regard to the imposition of financial penalties, it can be seen from the earlier figures that in this research it was a relatively infrequently used form of recommendation. In the case in which a financial penalty was recommended for a white offender, a process of reduction and elimination was used which led the reader towards the conclusion that a financial penalty was the most appropriate. After describing the previous probation experience as upsetting for the offender, the officer went on to cite the fact that the offender was in touch with both the educational welfare officer/schools social worker and the educational psychologist. The justification for excluding probation from the sentencing options was logical because there was a danger of the duplication of work.

Although there was no appreciable difference between the number of non-custodial recommendations for black and white offenders in the research, a number of significant qualitative differences were discernible. In four social-enquiry reports written on black offenders, reference was made in the conclusion and the final recommendation to a number of derogatory features directly attributable to the personality of the offender. Such comments did not tend to be present in accounts of white offenders. In one case a black offender is described in the recommendation as an:

> Amiable and able person, but these offences seem to have resulted from a rather passive and irresponsible attitude on his part. I think that they are indicative of his immaturity and of his inabilities to handle pressure appropriately. I believe that the time is right again to offer the support of supervision at this juncture. I have emphasised that the defendant will need to take the conditions of probation very seriously or face breach. He would also be expected to take part in an eight week preparation group for those newly placed on probation. I have considered another community service order, which the defendant himself feels negative about due to his previous experience. I should also add that I feel that at this stage there is a need for social work intervention.

The difference in the tone of this quotation is indicative of the qualitative difference found in reports on black offenders when compared with recommendations made for white offenders. Although the offender is described at the outset of the recommendation as 'amiable and able', the notion of the offender being a 'passive and irresponsible person' is introduced which has counterbalancing negative connotations. This impression is compounded by reference to his immaturity and inability to handle pressure appropriately. The suggestion that a probation order would be appropriate is followed by mention of a warning that has been made to the offender: he will face breach proceedings if he fails to take the probation order seriously. The effect of this is to raise doubts in the mind of the reader, particularly with regard to the possibility of the recommendation failing before the order has been made. The probability of a probation order being made must further have been reduced by mention of a 'negative' attitude towards community service and mention of the previous failure of a community-service order. Such a comment could possibly suggest to sentencers that the defendant himself would prefer a custodial sentence.

Surprisingly, the probation officer goes on to make his final recommendation in the following way:

A probation order with a condition of attendance at the Day Probation unit, is another sentence alternative under probation service control which appears to be the most relevant measure given his present situation. Such a groupwork programme would focus on his attitudes and behaviour in an extensive fashion. He has been seen in prison by a representative of the Day Probation unit and is acceptable in the unit.

One questions the credence that can be given to this recommendation, given the negative implications contained within the report relating to previous non-custodial intervention and that the defendant himself had expressed a desire not to be considered for a non-custodial sentencing option. The necessity for approaching the recommendation in this manner is unclear, but it was a distinctive feature in reports written on young black offenders. It would have been possible to have made this recommendation in a far more positive manner, as was the case in the reports written on white offenders. There was also a failure to address the issues which had been raised earlier in the report: the offender's problems at home and school, for instance. Although there was a recommendation for a non-custodial sentence, the force of the argument was reduced by both the inconsistencies within the argument and the negative context created within the recommendation.

In two instances some ambivalence was shown in the recommendation relating to black offenders when community service was being recommended which was not present in such recommendations made for white offenders. The following recommendation on a young black woman illustrates the point:

She presents as a bright intelligent person who is committed to the care of her child and of her family. She acknowledges the folly of her behaviour, and she is aware of her position before the court today. I have discussed with her and her family the various options which the court may consider. I believe that while a community service order may have something to offer her, in terms of reminding her firmly of the consequences of her behaviour, I feel that it would be difficult for her to maintain the commitment required due to her personal circumstances. I do believe however that as her offending is reaching a position in which she is becoming vulnerable and is in danger of jeopardising her freedom, there are social work tasks which could become useful to both her and her family and a short probation order would be a timely disposal.

A number of features within this recommendation distinguish it from similar statements relating to white offenders. The first section of the recommendation is positive: it is couched in a form of language acceptable to the courts. She is committed to her family, showing contrition by recognising the error of her ways and the gravity of the situation in which she finds herself. This offender was high within the 'tariff stakes': she had some five previous convictions against her which, as the probation officer acknowledges, put her in danger of a custodial sentence. There is then a possible danger in making a recommendation which is lower in the tariff, particularly since she appears to have been excluded from this option because of child-rearing commitments.

No examples were found of white offenders of either sex being excluded from any sentencing option on this basis, nor would black male offenders have been excluded for such a reason. The recommendation for probation does not appear to have been made with very detailed thought since the 'social-work tasks' are not delineated. In this case, then, it would seem that the offender suffers discrimination both as a young black person and as a woman. The recommendation is discriminatory and ill thought-out.

With regard to the imposition of financial penalties on young black offenders there appeared to be little qualitative difference. Non-recommendations were made in a number of cases in relation to black offenders. In one case the non-recommendation was couched in the following manner:

> I believe that I have given X a substantial number of chances to prove his motivation to see his order through and I can now reluctantly conclude that he is not ready for a probation order. In the light of the problems there have been in meeting the requirements of the probation order I do not feel able to offer any recommendation which involves willing cooperation with this service. I am aware that Mr X would leave custody with more rather than fewer problems and bearing in mind the four years when he avoided contact with the law, would respectfully suggest that should the court feel that custody is unavoidable, the experience be kept as brief as possible.

Although the probation officer's view that a non-custodial disposal is inappropriate in this case because of the offender's unwillingness to cooperate, the observation has to be made that such a negatively phrased form of recommendation was not found in any of the social-enquiry reports relating to white offenders.

The overall conclusion therefore is that probation officers presented arguments in relation to white offenders which were more credible to the courts in a number of respects. Social-enquiry reports tended to be couched in terms that were acceptable and understandable to the courts. The recommendations on white offenders also appeared to have a stronger internal logic than the recommendations on black offenders; they were more clearly related to the body of the report which also rendered them more readable, consistent and ultimately convincing. The absence of negative comments in reports on white offenders could indicate a greater enthusiasm to champion the cause of white offenders than black. It could also reveal a confusion on the part of probation officers on how to represent black offending appropriately.

QUALITATIVE DIFFERENCES BETWEEN PROBATION OFFICERS' ASSESSMENTS AND PROPOSED PRACTICE IN RELATION TO BLACK AND WHITE OFFENDING

In this section the relationship between the process of assessment in probation work and the proposed form of intervention will be examined comparatively with regard to black and white offenders. Within the literature there are a number of conceptualisations relating to social-work assessment. The lack of consensus in defining the nature of assessment even becomes apparent in the work of two writers, both of whom take the individual client as a starting point. Whittaker, for example, describes assessment in terms of a social-treatment model as:

> A joint process through which the worker and client explore and assess physical, psychological, and social conditions as they impinge on the client and then attempt to relate their findings to the range of social problems experienced by the client in a manner that yields objectives for change as well as a plan for action.
>
> (Whittaker 1974: 159)

Sheldon, writing from a more behavioural perspective, though nonetheless individualistic approach, emphasises that assessment is

inextricably linked to evaluation from the outset of all work with
social-work clients.

> Behavioural assessment is concerned with the identification of
> behaviours which it would be useful and reasonable to perform.
> Such assessment also takes into account the consequences of
> actions for all concerned in a social situation.
>
> (Sheldon 1982)

Both these views of assessment, although concentrating on judging
the 'client's' ability to function, encompass a wide variety of
activities which could be called social-work assessment. When
such diverse interpretations exist in the work of just two writers,
it is perhaps not surprising that individual probation officers who, it
will be argued, also start from an individualist perspective will also
have differing ideas on the nature of this central social-work task.

Much of the work carried out by the probation service is related
to assessment and plans for work related to those assessments.
Evidence for the way in which this process works will be drawn
from social-enquiry reports, interviews with probation officers and
records, part b and part c.

It was noteworthy that the initial assessments for all clients
appeared to be based upon highly individualised descriptions
of personality. This reflected the previously noted tendency of
probation officers to provide explanations of offending in terms
of individual and not societal causation. The subjective assessment
of the offender made by the probation officer usually formed the
basis for a suggested form of future social work. The nature of these
assessments was discretionary: the probation officer appeared to be
creating a certain form of reality which was meant to represent the
nature of the offender and the offender's problem.

In attempting to add to the understanding of the process of
assessment and planned intervention, data from interviews, social-
enquiry reports and part b and c records were examined. Evidence
was gathered about the possible relationship between assessment
and proposals for intervention from these sources for all 50
offenders.

One probation officer put the assessment and planning process
succinctly when in describing his work with an offender he said:

> I have no recognisable model, it has been a question of staggering
> from one appointment to the next.

This comment appeared to apply to much of the assessment and probation work examined in this research. Despite the *ad hoc* basis on which many of the officers appeared to operate, copious assessments were often present in the research.

Generally it was difficult to discern any generalised linkage between the form of the adjective used and the type of social-work intervention advocated. Many of the assessments seem to contradict the form of work advocated. There were a number of general qualitative differences in the way in which arguments were structured when assessments for black and white offenders were examined.

BLACK PHYSICALITY

The work of the West Midlands researchers in 1987 revealed an unusually high number of references to the physical presence of black offenders. In this research references to physicality were also frequently contained within the assessments on black offenders. The inclusion of such references was a significant distinctive factor which could lead to the conclusion that race is a factor in the assessment process. In one interview when a probation officer was asked to assess a black offender he described a:

Very physical presence . . . (pause) . . . he is a very dominant and strong personality, who is tall, very black and very handsome.

Frequently, as in the above case, the reference to physicality was followed by a reference to authority.

The officer continued:

His main problem is his relationship with authority. Despite his apparent dominance I suspect that he is very insecure. He also has a severe identity problem, and this means that he has to try and understand where he fits in. Although he comes down firmly as being black he has lost identification with his parents' generation, who were first generation West Indian, particularly his mother who does not conform to a stereotype. The overall problem is his finding a place in white society. He also grew up too quickly, he is still in fact nineteen. He is grown up physically, but he is still very much in his early teens. He hasn't matured much at all.

A number of important points emerge from this part of the interview. The probation officer himself appears to be highly aware of race and the blackness of this offender. It was the first point made in the verbal assessment and is heavily emphasised. Having acknowledged the offender's physicality the probation officer defines the 'problem' in terms of an inability to relate appropriately to authority. In the second interview the officer was asked to elaborate on this point. He did this by describing the offender's 'difficulties' as emanating from an inability to understand that:

> In this society at the end of the day, some people have power over you. There is nothing that you can do about that, X can't understand that.

The offender is also represented as being insecure, although at no point in the interview or in records was evidence given to support this part of the assessment. The reference to losing his identity is related directly to the offender's blackness and fitting in. This essentially assimilationist model, which was present in a number of black assessments, appears to assume that the offender will ultimately find identity and simultaneously desist from offending by assimilation into the dominant white society. The loss of identity is further compounded by the fact that the offender is estranged from his parents who were described as first generation. It is also noted by the probation officer that the mother in this case does not conform to a stereotype and while it could be read that the officer has an expectation that she should, it is important to note that mention of the stereotype followed reference to first generation black people.

The generation gap was mentioned by three other officers who also presented a stereotype of the first generation of parents characterised by quietism and passivity, who, according to probation officers, unlike their offending children were imbued with a work ethic. This factor in assessments was unique to black offenders. The last section of this assessment suggests that the root cause of this series of individual difficulties lies in the fact that the offender has not grown up. The argument in this assessment would appear to be as follows:

Three of these arguments – 1, 4 and 5 – are race-related, while the other two are based on the notion of the offender having a 'problem'. The last argument appears to lack a position in the

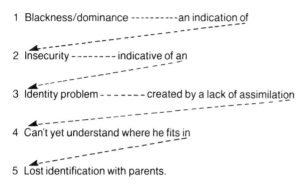

1 Blackness/dominance --------- an indication of

2 Insecurity -------- indicative of an

3 Identity problem ------- created by a lack of assimilation

4 Can't yet understand where he fits in

5 Lost identification with parents.

Figure 3.2   To show arguments used in assessments

development of the argument, possibly suggesting that there was some doubt on the part of the officer as to how this factor could be included. It is possible to see that even though the arguments relating to identity and insecurity are 'conventional' and can be seen in many assessments on white offenders, in the assessments on black offenders these conventional explanations are further complicated by the inclusion of race. The recommendation for practice which follows this assessment also includes a reference to race. The probation officer said:

> We have addressed the issue of racial harassment, it's been a difficult thing to verify, but I felt acknowledging his blackness was a positive step. I see the way to help him is to challenge certain racial stereotypes which have affected him. He feels aggrieved at being discriminated against.

This was as far as the analysis and associated form of intervention went. No indication was given by the officer as to how this challenge would or could happen. In this context it amounted to a statement of good intent which was not pursued in the work that followed. The question of a black offender's physicality was mentioned on other occasions in assessments and since it was found in previous research it needs to be examined more carefully. Four officers expressed an insecurity and inability in dealing with the physical blackness of offenders. For some officers a colour-blind approach would have been a simpler and more comfortable solution although there was a pervasive consciousness that suggested to officers that this might not be an appropriate response to the black presence. In a second interview the officer was asked to comment

on her previous spontaneously mentioned reference to physicality
with regard to a black offender. She said:

> I couldn't actually remember whether he is black or not, I don't
> really see him as black . . . (pause) . . . it wasn't until you
> mentioned that this client was black that I had thought of
> it. I'm afraid that this might be racist, I think that what we
> are being told is that there is no such thing as a recognisable
> race. Anyway for me he is very much a Laketown lad . . . a
> gentle giant, although there are flashpoints where he can get
> pretty nasty.

When the probation officer was questioned further about the
methods she would use, a one-to-one model was advocated. The
reason for this was described in terms of giving the offender the
space to look at his anger and enable him to take responsibility for
his actions. The probation officer was still advocating this course of
action despite the fact that in the social-enquiry report it was stated
that the offender had very little motivation and that probation had
little to offer this offender at the present time.

Although there were inconsistencies found in the kinds of arguments made in assessments and plans for social-work intervention
in the case of white offenders, the issue of racism appears further
to complicate already unclear issues. This seems to be related to
the inability and/or reluctance of probation officers to integrate a
black perspective into their assessments. Individualised assessments
are preferred and lead to a number of bewildering contradictions.

It becomes possible for a young black offender to be assessed
in the interview as being 'A girl, who had difficulty in relating
to people', while in the part b assessment she is described as
identifying quite strongly with black people and her racial identity.
In the interview and the records it emerged that this defendant
resisted 'group work' became of the fact that she has 'horror of
relating to people'.

The probation officer in the social-enquiry report had advocated
social-skills training in order to help the offender break down social
barriers which she created in interaction with people. It emerged in
the interview that there were other factors about the group which
the girl had objected to in that it was predominantly white and
male. This was not mentioned in any of the written material
and was a factor which the probation officer involved had not
thought necessary to mention in assessments. The question of

ethnic/racial identity was irrelevant, while the points that the offender was making about race and sex were apparently being ignored. Almost predictably the decision was made to work on a one-to-one basis with the probation officer in order to build up trust because this offender was unable to cope with the group. There was no explanation of how trust would be created and the ultimate benefit to the client of forming a trusting relationship with a white probation officer.

ASSESSMENT AND RACE

Probation officers appeared to experience problems in dealing with racism in assessments. Social-work methodology directed at black offenders was contextualised in a manner which was distinct from assessments of white offending, in that probation work was more likely to be directed at controlling the 'incredible amount of energy', or the 'almost hyper-active' black offender.

The most specific references made to race in assessments were in terms of the offender's relations with the police. In five cases, race was identified as influencing the way in which the officer would approach the 'case': a one-to-one form of work was advocated in which the offender would be encouraged with the officer to look at forms of self-protection and the way in which the offender deals with the police. In two of these cases the probation officer involved acknowledged the need to develop strategies to cope with racism. Police harassment of offenders was acknowledged in interview with probation officers, but was absent in assessments and social-enquiry reports despite the offender's own clearly stated view that racism was directly connected with his offending. Officers preferred to view the difficulties of intervention in terms of client idiosyncrasy:

It has proved difficult to focus the work that the offender has been doing, but what has emerged is X's attempts to channel all his considerable energy in a useful way that provides him with some satisfaction. He acknowledges that he finds it difficult to apply himself and often resorts to wandering around the town with friends which is what ultimately led him into trouble.

The validity of the offender's view of reality appears here to be diverted towards a conventional form of social-work reasoning which is likely to be more acceptable to the courts. This point relates to the previous work of Pinder, in a manner which both supports and refutes his findings. What is evident in this research is an absence of a coherent and explicit framework for recognising and representing specific racial and black identity, which is in keeping with Pinder's findings (Pinder 1984). In another important sense these findings stand in contradiction to Pinder when he argues that a failure to secure alternatives to custody and differential work with black offenders emanates from officers' recognition of the power of black offenders in stating their own interests and understandings. In this part of his work Pinder is making an important distinction between the needs of the offender and their interests. Thus a non-custodial sentence might fulfill a need: the offender is diverted from a potentially damaging experience of incarceration, while an anti-racist probation officer takes cognisance of a black offender's desire to put racism in the forefront of an assessment in an effort to represent the explanation of the offender. A probation officer, therefore, might take the offender's own view of police racial harassment and decide that given the view of the offender, probation intervention was impossible. This line of argument in Pinder's work could provide an explanation for differential forms of practice, but could be seen as good social-work practice in that the probation officer, by taking cognisance of the views of the offender, was attempting to practise in an anti-racist manner, even if this resulted in a custodial sentence. Thus the black offender's own view of reality is recognised and integrated into the probation officer/offender interaction. A different process appears to be occurring in this research, in that the probation officer appears to be attempting to ignore the offender's view of reality by diverting attention towards a form of personal abnormality, e.g. the excessive energy of the offender.

White offenders who were also described as being extremely energetic and outgoing were channelled into more conventional assessments, usually couched in terms of the white offender attending a probation group over eight weeks which would enable him to look closely at his offending and the circumstances surrounding that behaviour. Most importantly, it was more likely to be acknowledged in reports and interviews that white offenders accept the need for correction and acknowledge their foolishness, or, as one probation officer expressed it in a social-enquiry report on a white offender:

Accepts that it is important and timely to reconsider the direction in which he is heading, and I have impressed upon him the expectations of such an order. He is also aware that he would remain within the jurisdiction of the court should he commit a further offence during the current probation order.

In cases in which probation officers made favourable assessments of offenders, the fact that racism and the influence of race on the offence was not mentioned to the court resulted in the number of sentencing options being reduced since the required form of conventional argument acceptable to the court was not present. In interviews it was often clear that an offender's reluctance to accept forms of disposal, like community service and the day-probation programme, related to feelings about white society and white societal structures, particularly the criminal justice system. In one case the probation officer stated quite clearly in interview that the offender felt:

That it would be inappropriate for the 'client' to be associated with community service, even though he knew that the alternative might be custody.

Such feelings expressed by the offender were not recorded in the report, even though the explanation was given freely in the more informal interview setting.

What is stated above represents the general trend of the findings in relation to assessment. There were important exceptions to this. It was not always the case that probation officers preferred white offenders at a personal level. In comparing a probation officer's assessments on two young offenders, one black, one white, it was clear that the officer in question personally found greater rapport with the black offender than the white. The white offender was described in the part b records and in the interview as being isolated and defensive, with an arrogant manner. The black offender, however, was described as being likeable and outgoing. Once again, a reference was made to physicality in that he smiled a lot. The officer also saw him as being very cooperative. The one-to-one social-work method being used was very unproductive as far as the probation officer was concerned. The officer acknowledged that race was not raised as an issue at the point of assessment, although the offender felt victimised by the police. The officer felt it possible that he might see the probation service as being a part of white authoritarianism.

Here the dislike of the white offender's racism was expressed in the part c record as the following extract illustrates:

> I am finding it very difficult to engage X in anything mean-
> ingful. He rambles on at great length about peripheral matters,
> particularly his car, his comments are often bragging and racist.
> I sense a great degree of bitterness in him, perhaps deriving
> from his disability and this leads him to present himself in a
> very unattractive way.

In the interview it emerged that part of this unpleasant presentation was made manifest by a disability suffered by the white offender. The particular disability and the unpleasant personality, as far as the officer was concerned, combined together to make it quite difficult for him to work with this particular offender. A probation group was recommended in the social-enquiry report on the white offender as well as community service; a similar course of action was recommended for the black offender. The plan for probation work for the white offender reads as follows:

> While the court may be concerned that he was involved in
> offences involving a fifteen year old girl, nevertheless it is his
> first offence since 1979. My view is that he would be unlikely
> to re-offend in the near future whatever the outcome in the court
> here today, but a probation order may be of assistance in other
> respects.

The probation officer goes on to suggest a number of viable alternatives including community service and a fine – the latter disposal in the view of the officer being an acute punishment, since the offender normally manages his finances well. This should now be compared with the recommendation made for the likeable, outgoing black offender:

> These offences have arisen as a result of an irresponsible attitude
> on his part. I think that they are indicative of his immaturity and
> inability to handle pressure. Despite this it would be appropriate
> to offer the support of a supervision order, particularly at
> this time when he is about to attempt living on his own
> in accommodation found for him. Sending him out of the
> community would only delay his need to learn how to cope
> effectively within it. I considered another community service
> order, but feel that at this point there is a greater need for social

work intervention, particularly while he is feeling the pressure of his new environment.

In the last example the probation officer expressed a personal preference for working with the black offender; the plan for practice is presented in a far more positive way for the white offender. The officer makes a prediction that the white offender will not re-offend in the near future, which minimises any possible damage which might have been done by reference to the fact that these offences were committed with a fifteen-year-old girl. The positive factor relating to the fact that he can apparently manage his finances well is further positive proof of the viability of a non-custodial sentence.

The irresponsible attitude of the black offender referred to by the probation officer would not inspire the same confidence in a sentencer; neither would the difficulties experienced by the offender in handling the prospect of living alone. It is perhaps not surprising that the recommendation in the report was unacceptable to the courts. Officers during interview had difficulty in seeing their assessments and plans for action in the context of race and racism. All probation officers except one felt that race should only form part of the assessment if the question had a direct bearing on the commission of crime. There seemed to be variations, however, on what constituted 'direct bearing'. There was wide disagreement, for instance, as to whether the offender's personal views about race should be included in the assessment. Some probation officers seemed more happy to include race as a factor in assessment in the case, for instance, of racial abuse, but were less willing officially to record a black offender's anti-police feelings in an assessment.

No consensus emerged on any of these issues, only an ambivalence in attempting to place race within the context of assessment, social work intervention and plans. Some probation officers expressed an honest uncertainty about what was right and what was wrong with regard to the appropriate handling of young black offenders. There was an acknowledgement that 'culture' was in some vague manner significant, but probation officers had no way of knowing in what way this significance could be used in assessment and in the associated social-work intervention.

ASSESSMENT AND BLACK WOMEN

The question of gender is a crucial one since black women may be subjected to discrimination on the basis of gender (Walker 1985;

Worral 1990) and differential treatment related to racism. This general statement appears to apply to some black women offenders mentioned by probation officers in this study.

An observation that can be made about the question of gender and assessment is that officers wrote assessments on white women, which appeared to constitute a more detailed and sympathetic form of description than was the case with the black women offenders examined.[2] This point can be illustrated with reference to a white woman offender with a number of previous petty offences dating back to 1981. She was described by the white probation officer in the part b records as being quite prone to depression over some years, seemingly as a result of an insecure upbringing. As an adolescent she first identified with a group who used solvents and then with a group who used harder drugs. She was described as a:

> Pleasant intelligent young woman with a potential to make a positive life for herself, she is, however, unconfident and has a self-image badly in need of a boost, but she does not seem to respond to encouragement and attention.

The officer was most concerned with the offender's unresolved and ambivalent feelings for her mother. These offences seem to have been partly a 'vehicle for punishing her mother for not caring enough'. Money management, low motivation and the search for full-time work were other identified areas for concentration since the offender's debt is relatable to offending. Loneliness and over-emotional dependence, particularly on her close adult friends whom she regards as substitute mother-figures, were other target areas identified by the probation officer. The part b and c records indicated that all these areas were tackled, albeit in an *ad hoc* manner. Practical advice was given, particularly on the question of money management: the probation officer acted as a broker between hire-purchase companies, social security and the local council.

This degree of sensitivity was not present when the same probation officer was working with a young black woman who had very similar offences dating back to 1982. The part b records revealed that the probation officer had experienced difficulties in making initial contact with the offender and that she had made an effort to make her attend a probation group.

This offender was described as a very quiet woman who may find the group uncomfortable. The part b records indicated that she had failed to attend further interviews and despite the attempts made by the officer to reassure her that the group would be beneficial, it was not having any effect on the offender. It was also recorded that sessions between the probation officer and the offender were becoming unbearably uncomfortable and that the offender was unable to sit down and talk about her offending. It was difficult for the officer to create a constructive form of conversation, although this latter notion of constructive was not defined. In the interview the officer commented that the offender had not responded because of nervousness. After a number of months of interaction with her, the probation officer's assessment was that this offender was in a very vulnerable state, particularly with regard to her accommodation.

The officer went on to explain that the recommendation for probation was made on the understanding that the offender needed a basis for social skills, because she was very isolated, withdrawn and depressed. In the interview with the researcher, the officer was asked whether race was an important issue for this offender. The probation officer answered:

> I don't think it was an issue. It certainly hasn't been a regular focus for our discussions, it has come up, the problem being that she is so inarticulate that she's unable to explain her feelings about this. The overriding thing about her is her susceptibility, she tends to always say what you want her to say and you can get any answer out of her you want, whatever you want her to say she will say. When I have gone to her flat it didn't look to me that there was much white influence about, she had a big poster on the wall which pertained to be about back home, but I am unable to comment on that. I suppose it did look on reflection that she was trying to identify quite strongly with being black. The problem really is that I feel she has no sense of herself, or who she is. I want to give her some feeling of belonging. I don't think that she's got that, and I feel if I'm going to be a good social worker I should recognize the fact that her experiences earlier of this mixed cultural experience must be significant, and that not belonging is a problem. Yes, I think that I am quite embarrassed about it, I feel terribly uncertain about what's right and what's wrong. If I was supposed to be a white liberal who is open to these things I feel really hampered by not knowing. There is a feeling that there is a right and a wrong, and I am very unclear what is right and what is wrong.

This is a significant view and has been quoted at length since it reflects the idea that not belonging to the dominant culture lies at the root of this offender's identity problem. It would appear to exemplify an assimilationist position, since the task of a good social worker is to enable the offender to develop a feeling of belonging to the dominant culture. It is also important to note that having made this point, the officer shows some confusion as to what is right and wrong in this context.

The above quotation is also remarkable in the way it attempts to underestimate the offender's attempts to identify with her own blackness. The picture on the wall in the flat would seem to have significance to the offender, but was given cursory attention by the officer. The overriding concern was with the vulnerability and female hopelessness which the officer saw as being central to the problems experienced by the young woman.

The white probation officer was able to identify a clear role with the white offender discussed earlier, and could appreciate her as being pleasant and attractive. White women offenders tended to be presented as being under considerable stress, having suffered as a result of a combination of events that were beyond individual control. The form of social work that was most usually advocated was that of one-to-one casework. The justification for this was that this form of work could assist the offender in making decisions.

This contrasts with the way in which black women offenders were frequently described in terms of being impoverished, nervous and taciturn. Problems in the family were also more likely to be mentioned in relation to black women offenders than white. The social work based on this assessment was recommended in more general terms, although it usually involved some form of one-to-one casework with the offender. For white women offenders, what appeared to emerge when assessments and plans for action were examined were conventional forms of assessment and action which constituted a predictable form of argument. A conventional assessment on a white woman could be related to the conventional form of explanation mentioned in Chapter 1 and is described in Figure 3.3.

This form of probation reasoning, linking assessment with proposed practice, did not apply to black women offenders, although the social-work methods were roughly comparable in that one-to-one work was recommended. The bases for reaching the conclusion that casework was most appropriate for black women offenders were different and unconventional. Thus the 'genuinely inadequate' white woman was not applicable to the assessment of the black offender. In assessments on white women it was far more likely to see 'A cry for help from a very troubled young woman'. These cries for help were not as evident in assessments on black women offenders. The intrinsic worth of the social-work relationship and the power of the relationship in itself to create beneficial results, although present in assessments on black women, were not argued with the same enthusiasm. In this research there was some evidence to suggest that black women were also having the experience of being black denied them by both white men and women probation officers. Unlike the 'vulnerable' white women involved with probation, black women were conceptualised as suffering from a peculiarly 'feminine' form of 'silliness'.

A COMPARATIVE EXAMINATION OF DAILY PROBATION PRACTICE UNDERTAKEN WITH BLACK AND WHITE OFFENDERS

The justifications in records and social-enquiry reports frequently revolved around the notion of providing the offender with the opportunity of examining his offending behaviour. Nothing was said about the form which this examination would take. It seemed to be assumed by probation officers that offenders had not previously been through this process of examination. It was

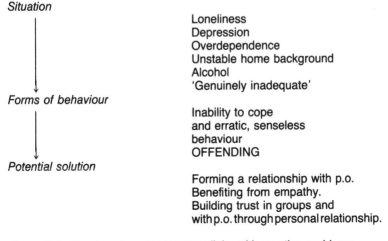

Situation

Loneliness
Depression
Overdependence
Unstable home background
Alcohol
'Genuinely inadequate'

Forms of behaviour

Inability to cope
and erratic, senseless
behaviour
OFFENDING

Potential solution

Forming a relationship with p.o.
Benefiting from empathy.
Building trust in groups and
with p.o. through personal relationship.

Figure 3.3   To show how assessment links with practice problems

not possible to find any explanation of the benefits of this process for the offender. The proposition seems to be made here that it might be possible to reduce offending behaviour through a process of self-examination in which the inherent foolishness of offending would be understood. The aim appeared to be applicable to both black and white offenders.

Many of the tasks performed by probation officers related to practical problems which could occasionally be described as crisis intervention. An example of such work most frequently cited in this research was the non-arrival of a benefit giro cheque. When probation officers were questioned on this aspect of their work in interviews, they seemed to regard this as secondary to the formulation of a social-work relationship. This finding is similar to that of Fielding's study which reported that probation officers, although frequently engaging in work of a practical nature as they attempt to assist in the resolution of personal practical difficulties, do not define it as central to probation work (Fielding 1984).

No evidence was found to indicate a greater or lesser willingness on the part of probation officers to assist black offenders with such practical difficulties. Probation officers in this work offered many forms of practical help to both black and white offenders on a daily basis which included negotiation with various government departments, most notably in relation to social-security payments, domestic budgeting, assistance with the securing of employment and negotiations regarding debt. Four probation officers stated that they felt black offenders were less willing than white offenders to ask for this kind of help from the probation service. Black offenders, unlike many of their white contemporaries, tended to allow situations to develop in uncontrollable ways before asking for help.

On 16 occasions practical difficulties developed into major crises and detailed records were found of such situations in the part c records. Crises developed in a number of areas that were common to black and white offenders. They were in the area of finances in which debts, including the non-payment of fines, appeared to be a threat to the liberty of the offender. Davies has defined the goals of crisis intervention as:

> Counteracting the effects of a crisis, to relieve the symptoms of emotional pain, and to restore the client to a state of being able to function normally.

(Davies 1985:171)

It was the case in the records that officers were able to respond swiftly and imaginatively to specific problems that were placed before them. Significantly in these interactions black and white offenders were passive parties to the negotiations. Thus officers 'took over' responsibility in crises and appeared to be reasonably successful in assisting offenders in the short term. Seven male white offenders and three white women offenders experienced crises and were assisted by the supervising probation officer, while only three black male and three black women offenders were recorded as experiencing crises.

Group work was another form of social-work intervention which was undertaken with a number of offenders and this was of varying types. It is necessary at this point to give a brief account of the forms of group-work practice which were established at the time the research was carried out. The daily programme organised by the Laketown service provided the opportunity for sentencers to make probation orders with a special condition requiring the offender to attend a programme organised by the service for a ten-week period four days a week at the beginning of the order. Legal authority for such a condition is contained within the Criminal Justice Act 1982. The facility was specifically designed for offenders who, at severe risk of a custodial sentence. These group sessions, of one and a half hours duration, were designed to 'focus clearly' on offending behaviour, its causes and consequences, both in general and for the individual member in particular, for their families and the victims of the offences. Social skills and group-work methods were used to 'help clients explore their offending behaviour in some depth and detail'.

There was no indication that this form of provision was being differentially utilised by probation officers. In all cases in which probation was being recommended and an offender was in the 'high tariff' risk group, the programme was recommended. Formal groups were also run for new probationers: the introduction to probation group was designed to 'Help clients assess together their reasons for offending'. The alcohol group aimed at 'confronting offenders' who had been in trouble through alcoholic drink. The majority of offenders attended these groups as a condition of the probation order.

Much of the recorded material on day-to-day interactions within these and other groups was kept by key workers. In some cases it appeared that black offenders were more willing to communicate with white probation officers in a group. Accounts of black offenders in custody reveal that they frequently took a prominent part in discussions, occasionally taking the opportunity to voice views relating to racist features of the institutional regime. Black women offenders particularly found it difficult to relate to others in groups. When this occurred it was likely to be interpreted as an inadequacy on the part of the offender. Two black offenders specifically voiced objections to being in a group with white offenders. It was difficult to find material which reflected the experience of black and white offenders comparatively in group sessions. A number of questionnaires were discovered, however, relating to the offenders' own assessment of the probation programme. Answers were found by one black male offender and one white male offender. The questions and answers for both black and white offenders were as follows:

1 What was the group about?
   White response: Rehabilitation.
   Black response: I don't know.

2 What have you enjoyed about the group?
   White response: I have enjoyed the debate.
   Black response: Nothing.

3 Is there anything you would like to change about your situation?
   White response: I'd like to find somewhere to live.
   Black response: I'd like a job.

4 Is there anything you would like to change about yourself while on probation; if so, what?
   White response: A little more organisation would be handy, self-discipline.
   Black response: Nothing.

5 Think about the following areas of your life. Tick any that you may need help with while on probation.

Family relationships.	White response: OK.
	Black response: Nothing.
Partners	White response: This is not the business of the Social Services.
	Black response: OK.
Alcohol	White response: No problem.
	Black response: No problem.

6 Do you think that probation can help with this; if so, why?

White response: Advice, etc.

Black response: Blank.

7 What is your personal agenda for the future?
White response: Job, drama college, writing, fame, parties, and
an early retirement to somewhere hot where I could waste my
life in comparative comfort.
Black response: Blank.

Although it is very difficult to draw any conclusions on the basis
of two completed questionnaires, it seemed that the white offender
was more integrated into the group than the black offender. The
black offender's response seems to have been one of indifference:
the records indicated that he attended the group on sufferance and
that breach had been threatened if he did not attend. A clear message
that did appear from the questionnaire was that the black offender
wanted a job.

The responses given by the white offender suggest a willingness
to give what he perceives to be appropriate responses. It may also
have been possible that this offender did, for instance, enjoy some
of the debates, as was indicated by his recognition of the need for
more self-discipline. There was an apparent inability on the part
of the black offender to see any benefit in what was being offered
by the probation service. In other words the blank responses were
very powerful statements in that they pose questions relating to the
viability of using methods that had been developed in social-work
textbooks and training courses dominated by white people.

PROBATION OFFICERS' EVALUATION OF THEIR
WORK WITH BLACK AND WHITE OFFENDERS

The idea of evaluation in practice relates to the phase of work
in which the extent to which social-work objectives have been
realised is assessed. Sheldon, a behaviourist, argues that evaluation
should occur throughout the social-work process and emphasises
the importance of the specificity of goals and the establishment
of baselines for problem behaviour prior to intervention. This,
he argues, makes the task of measurement considerably easier.
Although this method of evaluation provides tangible evidence of,
for instance, improved functioning in a specific area of behaviour,
situations faced by offenders are multi-faceted, which makes the
problem of selecting one particular behavioural pattern for attention

almost impossible. Indeed, one of the major problems facing probation officers in this research was the complex nature of diffused client goals. Browne has argued that, in practice, very few structured approaches similar to that advocated by Sheldon and other writers are used in day-to-day practice. Even when they are used the terminology is not understood, the theory not employed and the structure imprecise (Brown 1978).

One of the major problems in using such models is that they require considerable time, since methods of recording evaluative data have to be developed and recorded. Such processes will often involve negotiating with another individual in order to monitor the process. It should be stressed that time-limited, structured interventions like the task-centred model appear to be relatively instrumental in the creation of changed offender-behaviour patterns. Work carried out by a number of researchers indicates that when social work is evaluated, a task-centred approach in controlled comparisons appears to have positive effects on clients' social and interpersonal problems, leading to a reduced need for social and psychiatric services (Goldberg 1977).

One of the important observations relating to structured methods is that the 'client's' problem is focused upon for work, which tends to deflect attention from the part played by macro-structural problems like unemployment, which is frequently beyond the offender's control. Mention of such evaluated methods, and indeed any formal social-work methodology, was virtually absent from accounts given by probation officers. Probation officers when interviewed tended to talk about the offender's future or the past in anecdotal terms. Records were usually written descriptions of life events containing little evidence of formal evaluation of social-work intervention on black or white offenders.

Very broad statements which can be described as evaluative were found in some 15 of the cases which were examined and tended to be undetailed and usually made in relation to black offenders rather than white. The part b records contained most evaluative statements, although these comments tended to be impressionistic in that they recorded improvements in attitude to work or a greater level of maturity. No effort was made to break down dysfunctional behaviours into their constituent parts, to prioritise problems and then to work at each problem area as suggested by Sheldon and other writers. Statements relating to evaluation made in interviews were also vague.

On occasions work was evaluated in social-enquiry reports and although recommendations have been examined in a previous section the evaluation in this aspect of work needs to be examined separately. These attempts at evaluation were usually subsumed under the heading 'response to supervision'. Responses were evaluated in descriptive terms. X showed an 'erratic response'. Y's improvement was conceptualised in terms of development of trust. No indication was given as to the meaning of terms like trust. The intermediate treatment group was described as having mixed success although the nature of the success is not elaborated. Records were examined in an attempt to understand the meaning the officer was ascribing to success. No further reference appeared to be made to evaluation or successful practice in any of the material examined. Overall, this assessment of response to supervision lacked clarity which makes any evaluation of the work carried out extremely difficult. The probation officer appears to be reporting a partial success in that support and guidance was provided to the offender at the period between school and work, although this was not sufficient to keep the offender out of trouble.

The problems in using reconviction rates in evaluating probation work have been discussed within the social-work literature. Reconviction rates for juveniles and young offenders receiving custodial sentences are published annually by the prison department. Sixty-six per cent of those released from youth custody are reconvicted within two years. Some 47 per cent of adult prisoners and 40 per cent of probationers are reconvicted within two years (Home Office 1988a). It is difficult to draw any meaningful conclusion from reconviction rates, since populations are regionally different in respect of age structures, criminal histories and offending patterns. Reoffending may also measure the effectiveness of policing in different areas. Changes in offending behaviour cannot be described in such simple terms. A comparative appraisal of the different forms of intervention and their effectiveness in preventing reoffending is further hampered by the fact that few studies deal with offending histories. Writers have argued that the defendant's criminal history and current living situation outweigh the type or length of any intervention in determining the likelihood of reconviction (Rutter and Giller 1983). These figures seem to have been unchanged by the new, tougher regimes in detention centres (NACRO 1987). This research suggests that probation officers' notion of success is related directly to the development of a relationship with an offender, rather than any tangible effects that the intervention might have had in terms of preventing black and white offenders from being reconvicted. 'Talking through problems' was an activity which was seen as being intrinsically worthwhile. Officers did not see any problems with this orientation to their work, since this had been the prevailing orthodoxy on training courses and was the form of work expected by the probation service. When the question of reconviction rates as a possible measure of success was approached, probation officers seemed bewildered. They replied with an unequivocal rejection of the idea for both black and white offenders. One probation officer summed up the view expressed by most of the officers interviewed when he was asked:

Q.   Do you think that you can use reconviction rates as a measure of success of a probation order?

A.   No, I certainly don't . . . forming a relationship with a probation officer can do far more than one can measure in such a crude way. Often you can build up trust. Often you can give the offender space to say the kinds of things he has never been able to say to anyone else. Often you can help the person come to terms with problems. You can also identify problems that have not been identified before.

Most probation officers interviewed defined success either in terms of establishing a relationship with offenders, as was stated above, or diverting offenders away from custodial sentence. Probation and the achievement of the probation order when a custodial sentence was probable was also seen as a form of successful intervention. More attention was directed at success in the context of getting a recommendation accepted by a sentencer than in the actual form of the intervention that followed.

In accepting these two criteria of success as defined by probation officers, it would appear that black offenders in this small sample were disadvantaged on both counts. First, probation officers despite a recommendation for non-custody were less likely to be successful in diverting a black offender from custody. Second, the white probation officer will experience other difficulties in forming relationships with black offenders. Thus in the terms applied by probation officers, work with black offenders is less successful.

Chapter 4

Language, power and convention

In previous chapters the sequencing of arguments and the acceptance or non-acceptance of explanations contained in probation officers' reports was examined with reference to the social construction of black and white crime. This chapter is concerned with the elements of such explanations: the combination of words into the discourse that frames social-work knowledge and authority, confirming differential 'client' status on black people. Rojek and Collins have described the importance of the concept of discourse in the following way:

> In working with people social workers use words and character-istic forms of impression management. These forms and words correspond to specialised systems of knowledge regarding the subjects and object of social work. They refer to a specific discourse, a specific way of organising meaning and establishing authority. Learning to be a social worker may be in part, a matter of being seen as competent in the received professional language and knowledge.
>
> (Rojek and Collins 1988: 613)

During the 1970s and early 1980s Marxists of various complexions attempted to demonstrate how social work reproduces capitalist class relations through state agencies like the probation service, while pluralists utilised rehabilitative models, emphasising the need to work within existing social structures (Corrigan and Leonard 1978; Davies 1985; Walker and Beaumont 1985). By concentrating on the activities that constitute probation work – speaking and writing – this chapter aims to extend these theoretical debates with specific reference to the way in which black people are treated by the probation service.

THE USE OF OTHER LANGUAGES

The use of creole has a symbolic connection with the slavery plan-
tation and is conceptualised by some writers as being a bedrock for
the foundation of a black-youth culture which resists institutional
racism. Some black people conceptualise creole in terms of a
defensive esoteric form of communication which excludes white
people (Cashmore 1979; Hebdige 1976). During the 1970s the creole
of black youth came to be referred to as 'dread talk', dread being
defined by Hewitt as:

> Worthy of respect as an initiate of a black Jamaican cultural
> mystery the indicators of which were a commitment to reggae
> music, the employment of creole, and an assiduously maintained
> separation from intercourse with white people.
>
> (Hewitt 1986: 101)

The importance of creole decreased during the 1970s, when the
word dread came to convey a more general meaning: in Hewitt's
words it was 'simply equated with good'. The creole languages
utilised by black people in Britain vary from French-based patois
(Dominica and St Lucia) to the Guyanese 'Bajan' (Barbados) and
other forms of patois deriving from other Caribbean islands. The
Jamaican creole has been substantially analysed by a number of
writers. Hewitt makes an important distinction between the creole
of those who were socialised in Jamaica and those brought up in
England who utilise creole with English. Estimates of the extent
to which British-born black people use creole vary widely. Some
research claims that some 95 per cent of black children speak
some creole while other studies find lower proportions ranging
between 10 and 20 per cent of young black people utilising
creole in everyday speech. Hewitt concludes that young black
people in London do not use creole constantly, but tend occasionally to use patois forms with strong Jamaican pronounciation
(Hewitt 1986).

If the use of creole can be associated with the development of a
form of cultural separatism, we might have expected this to be a
feature of resistance to probation intervention. The use of creole
was not reported by probation officers in research carried out in
1989, although the small sample size would make it impossible
to draw any firm empirical conclusions from this finding. Work
carried out in the mid-1970s did suggest that probationers were

'breaking into creole' in order to confuse and possibly resist the probation officer (Denney 1976).

Children are frequently called upon by probation officers to 'translate' when parents have little English. This can be problematic for parents who may not wish children to know everything about a specific problem. When a black probationer is fluent in English, some first-language features are carried through into the second language, with the placing of different emphases on words within a sentence. Difficulties in translation are not simply a matter of accent and idiom, but also the creation of linguistic frameworks which have no English equivalent. (For a full account see Ely and Denney 1987.)

PREVIOUS LITERATURE

Attempts have been made in the literature to analyse linguistic interactions between probation officers and offenders, mostly in the form of recordings and observations of the spoken word in interviews, although few of these studies have included any discussion of racism (Goldberg and Stanley 1985; Willis 1986; Day 1981). Some feminist analyses of the criminal justice system have been more successful in deconstructing differential forms of treatment administered to women by the courts and welfare agencies like the probation service (Allen 1987; Worral 1990).

An important distinction has been made by Rodger in attempting to define the analysis of social-work discourses. There is the project that studies the construction of different knowledges and power within social-work interactions and the ethnomethodological project of studying how knowledgeable human beings build up and negotiate meaning through social interaction (Rodger 1991).

Carlen (1976), using both forms of analysis in her analysis of the language of magistrates' courts, demonstrated how notions of 'common sense' were invoked by sentencers and other court officials in order to create 'self-evident truths'. Carlen draws on Heidegger to argue that:

> Common sense has its own necessity; it extracts its due with the weapon appropriate to it, namely an appeal to the 'self-evident' nature of its claims and considerations.
>
>   (Heidegger 1949, quoted in Worral 1990: 19)

The criminal justice system, as Carlen argues, is governed by personnel, some of whom are given authority to define others. The probation officer's common sense, which is claimed to be universally recognisable by those who use it, is a 'specific discourse sanctioned by law' and as Worral argues 'elevated in practice to the status of expertise' (Worral 1990: 18).

In a recent ethnomethodological research project Stanley was concerned to understand the procedures which ordered probation officer/'client' interactions. He found that topics initiated by probation officers were initially met with responses that did not signify immediate acceptance by the probationer. Despite this, Stanley illustrates how the probation officer, through a complex repertoire of responses, is empowered to initiate, continue or terminate topics of conversation (Stanley 1991). Although this research assists in understanding the sequencing of linguistic interaction between probation officer and offender, it is to the way in which knowledge is constituted and transmitted through language that attention is now directed.

STRUCTURALIST ANALYSIS AND PROBATION INTERVENTION

Although structuralism has been considered by social-work theorists during the 1980s (Rojek *et al.* 1988; Rodger 1991) there is little available evidence to suggest that such conceptualisations have been regarded by social-work practitioners as utilisable or relevant concepts. Movements in analytical method present a number of possibilities for the understanding and enhancement of probation work with black people. It will not be possible in this short chapter to present anything like an adequate explanation of the significance of these concepts to practice, or to present more than a brushstroke account of the central ideas.

It is in the field of discourse analysis that we are most likely to find a clearer understanding of the way in which professional language is constructed. Some structuralist theorists, most notably Saussure, argue that there is a relation between the sentence and discourse, in as much as there are forms of organisation that order all linguistic systems which give them meaning.

The basic premise of structuralist analysis can be illustrated in Figure 4.1 where it can be seen that the sentence and meaning are linked through the mediation of discourse. Words are not symbols that correspond to referents since there is an arbitrariness which lies at the heart of language. It is the systematic relationship between words that enable them to communicate, rather than the relationships between words and things. Language is not an instrument for reflecting a pre-existent reality, since subjects are produced by linguistic structures (Selden 1989). Saussure defined the verbal sign or word as the union of the signifier, that is, the sound or written symbolisation of a sound, and the signified, which is the concept. There is therefore no reason why cat should denote a feline quadruped, as Lodge puts it, since the English language would work equally well if cat and dog changed places in the system, as long as all users were aware of the change (Lodge 1981).

Selden uses the example of traffic lights to illustrate the point. Red is the signifier while stop is the signified. Red denotes stop, while connoting danger. Elements of language acquire meaning not as a connection between words and things, but as part of a system of relations (Selden 1989).

What we are most interested in here is the use of terminology and language in the probation officer's discourse. It is clear that the different levels of meaning reside both within the words used and beyond them. An important set of distinctions is offered by Saussure and are referred to in the literature as 'langue' and 'parole'. Langue is the linguistic system that we learn from a language (Saussure 1974). An example of this system would be the basic rules governing the conjugation of verbs in any language. Parole denotes the way in which speech is used in everyday life, the innumerable utterances spoken in language which might not always adhere to the basic rules of a language. The diversity and complexity of meanings within parole are shown in relation to the way in which probation officers develop a quasi-professional terminology, as, for instance, when they talk of creating boundaries for clients or creating space.

The parole of probation can best be described as the 'signification' of the offender to the court or other official bodies like the courts through the medium of legal instruments, e.g. social-enquiry

Figure 4.1   To show basic premise of discourse analysis

reports. A semiological analysis of this form of parole enables us to attempt to deconstruct the innumerable utterances spoken and written within the discourse to the courts, the social-enquiry report or the probation record.

Probation officers and black people should not be seen simply as inactive victims of imposed ideological constructs. Attention should be directed towards the signification of meanings through competing discourses. The complexity of the use of one word in a report can be used to illustrate the point. In the following report on a white offender the probation officer, after cataloguing the 'unstable' home background, wrote:

> X is the youngest of four children. Her parents divorced in 1975 after a long period of marital disharmony. Part of my supervision with her has concentrated on helping her to come to terms with residual ambivalent feelings towards her mother, by whom she has felt rejected over the years.

This extract could have denoted to the magistrate an offender who has been a victim of family problems and yet the connotations could possibly project not only a past problem but a future solution, which in one sense makes the offender eligible for acceptance into the realms of clientisation. A key to the image of the offender is held in the term 'disharmony', a word close to its antonym harmony and could therefore infer the possibility of harmony in this particular case. The report also gives evidence of harmony between the probation officer and 'client' in dealing with her feelings towards her mother, which could also be seen as inferring a future harmony between the offender and her mother. Once this family harmony is achieved there is an implication that the offending will cease, since it was a disharmony that apparently caused the offending in the first place. Yet what is the connotative value of terms such as harmony and disharmony? There a possible musical connotation is created in which more than one instrument creates a unified sound. It is this unity that would seem to be the solution to the 'client's' offending. What then is the nature of this unity? From the report it would seem to be threefold. The desired unity of:

1 Mother and father.
2 Probation officer and 'client'.
3 'Client' and mother.

What holds these three pairs together is an idea of the possible unity and harmony of one individual with another. Such unity is presented as being achievable by the probation officer and the result is harmonic, musical and desirable. With time and practice and the orchestration of the probation officer, all will lead to harmony. A probation order could provide the necessary conditions conducive to this creation.

The term 'disharmony' is also used in an explanation of black offending when the probation officer writes:

> The records indicate a turbulent and violent home background. His father's marriages have been characterised by disharmony and violence. Perhaps this violent background goes some way to explaining the number of offences of aggression.

Here the possible connotative value of the term 'disharmony' already given is negated by the use of the word 'violence'. The image of the musical and potentially melodic is severely qualified by the use of the term violence. The disharmony is seen as being connected with marriages which have been characterised by the use of violence. While on the surface these two explanations for offending are the same for both the black and white offender – i.e. the family disharmony – the connotations of the social-enquiry report on the black offender has an additional dimension. Violence is something that threatens harmony. No indication is given of any change in the father's behaviour. The violence that has been persistent, in that all his marriages have been characterised by violence, connotes an unceasing disharmony. What is interesting when the use of this term is compared in the two cases is that we do not know the nature of the disharmony in the white parental situation and yet this potentially damaging extra information was thought appropriate to include in this report by the probation officer in relation to the black offender.

What then is the connotational value of the term 'violence' which is repeated twice in the space of two lines, and is connected with the term turbulent? It has negative connotations of uncontrollable behaviour and may invoke images which are associated with the unpredictable and the destructive. Therefore in the first social-enquiry report that used the term disharmony the overall picture could be perceived as unifying while in the case of the report on the black offender there is an association with wild destruction although both extracts are written within a form of social-work discourse.

POST-STRUCTURALIST DEVELOPMENTS[1]

Saussure's claim to have embarked on a science of signs is often 'dismissed as a hopeless ambition' by some current social-work theorists (Rojek *et al.* 1988). It has to be acknowledged that Saussure's work does constitute an important basis for under-standing the nature of professional discourses.

Sibeon argues that pro-Saussurian theories of language imply that there are no possibilities of discursively redefining and changing social work:

> The central methodological implication of structuralist linguis-tics is that, because language has an underlying structure of its own, and because speech (parole) is derived from language (langue) and given meaning by it in ways beyond the conscious grasp of human actors, the study of (social work) knowledge should never begin with the micro situational study of speech instances (parole) but instead should begin with the study of social langue as a whole, i.e. as a 'deep' autonomous and objec-tively 'real' facticity that exists independently of its situational expressions.
>
> (Sibeon 1991: 29)

Saussure recognised that the signified and the signifier constituted two systems, but, having conceptualised language as a system independent of physical reality, retained the coherence of the sign. Post-structuralist theorists, as Selden argues, attempt to 'prise apart' the two halves of the sign in order to understand the changing nature of the signifier:

> Structuralist critics set out to master the text and to open out its secrets. Post-structuralists believe that this desire is vain because there are unconscious, or linguistic, or historical forces which cannot be mastered.
>
> (Selden 1989: 109)

The proposition that the meaning of things has a structural basis in language suggests that terms used by probation officers like 'boundary' or 'counselling' have no specific meaning, since the meaning of words derives from their structural position in the language system of which they form a part. The relationship between signifier and signified is not universal. The word 'contract' is currently used in probation practice to describe a verbal agreement or written document which denotes the rules of engagement and goals to be achieved within an 'agreed' timeframe. The probation order is in one sense a contract: the probation officer is required to advise, assist and befriend the offender, who in turn is required to comply with statutory requirements such as allowing the probation officer to visit his home and reporting to the probation officer when required. The idea of a contract forms the basis for much task-centred casework in probation, although the probation officer has a range of sanctions that can be used against the offender in the event of non-compliance, the most radical being the breach proceeding. Having been convicted, the probationer does not have recourse to any official mechanisms in the event of her/him having a grievance against the probation officer. The contract cannot constitute binding obligations on both sides since one of the parties, the probation officer, has legal powers of redress in the event of the agreement breaking down which the other party, the offender, does not possess. The signifier 'contract' connotes differential meanings and obligations depending on the access to power within the criminal justice system (Rojek *et al.* 1988).

The competing nature of discourses determines what is possible and impossible to say in a social-enquiry report. Instead of reconstituting what Foucault calls 'chains of inference', as we have already seen in probation discourse, probation officers should be aware of the systems of dispersion. Foucault describes such systems in terms of a series of 'gaps', intertwined with one another, interplays of differences, distances and substitutions (Foucault 1972). The reader of social-enquiry reports is confronted with:

> Concepts that differ in structure and in the rules governing their use, which ignore or exclude one another, and which cannot enter the logical architecture.
>
> (Foucault 1972: 37)

POWER AND 'PROFESSIONAL' LANGUAGE

In earlier attempts to analyse probation discourse, concentration was focused upon the spoken word (Willis 1986; Stanley 1991). In post-structuralist forms of analysis the distinction between the written and the spoken is problematic and for our purposes no clear distinction will be made. Discourses are constructed by 'clients' and welfare professionals; inequitable power relationships often revolve around the competing nature of the discourses involved in probation work. While self-evident truths and common sense constitute a powerful discourse, the formulation of 'technical' concepts presupposes the existence of a shared system of specialist meanings constituting a technical form of discourse removed from the language of the 'client'. Probation officers use concepts both among themselves, in official documents, and in conversations with 'clients' in such a way as to suggest agreed meanings, which could be shared with other professionals within the criminal justice system.

The meanings associated with notions of 'boundary' and 'space' exemplify the interface of quasi-technical concepts, codes and institutionalised processes. In the research described in earlier chapters, the creation of boundaries was frequently advocated in 'counselling' work, which was primarily concerned with problems perceived by probation officers to be connected with personal relationships. The probation officer refers to a white woman as:

> An intelligent person who has never had difficulties in opening up in our sessions, although keeping to a regular reporting pattern, centred her not only on the crisis but also on issues between us at times. She does respond much better now to the firm boundaries which I try to place on supervision, and she is able to acknowledge why it is important for her even though she resents the boundaries.

Here the officer moves through the following sequence of discursive units:

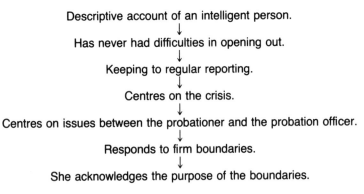

Descriptive account of an intelligent person.
↓
Has never had difficulties in opening out.
↓
Keeping to regular reporting.
↓
Centres on the crisis.
↓
Centres on issues between the probationer and the probation officer.
↓
Responds to firm boundaries.
↓
She acknowledges the purpose of the boundaries.

Figure 4.2   To show sequence of discursive units

Not unusually, throughout this passage the reader is confronted with a complex of differentiated concepts, connected by gaps of inference. The notion of the probationer being 'intelligent' is linked to 'opening out', which could refer to an ability to articulate. In expressing the interaction in terms of centring the subject's problems encapsulated in the word 'crisis', the officer widens the discursive formation to include issues between the officer and client. The boundary does not constitute the beginning of a new paragraph, but follows the previous sentence which may suggest a linkage between issues and boundaries. The boundaries are firm and resented by the probationer although the officer deduces that the probationer is able to see the need for their introduction.

The boundary appeared to contain a legitimating quality conferring firmness and structure on the intervention, while simultaneously producing a contradictory response in the probationer who resented the boundary but understood the purpose of its imposition. This prompted the researcher in a second interview to ask the officer what was meant by the term boundary in the context of the above quotation:

> It's about not letting the client go too far, holding on to what is, keeping them within the realms of reality.

Boundary in this case, then, seemed to suggest to the officer a centring of reality orientation within the casework relationship. Other officers appeared to be using the term in connection with legal boundaries in relation to acceptable behaviour while on probation and the possibility of breach proceedings or boundaries in relationships with others. What is important here is that such a term was used in official probation records in such a way as to suggest that there is a common understanding about the meaning of the term boundary, since the word remained unqualified in all forms of material examined. It has to be acknowledged that there are a number of ways in which the boundary concept can be used within sociological theory. Following Durkheim, Erikson has argued that the principle underlying the argument is that people need boundaries, and that without clear guides for action people discover these effective boundaries by deviance (Erikson 1966). Fielding has argued in his study of probation practice:

> In arguing for boundaries probation officers are discovering in the client centred ideology how control can be presented as need. The control work that they are obliged to perform,

can be justified by the discovery of people's need for boundary defining.

(Fielding 1984: 48)

The subject is in 'the process of becoming' the 'good subject' who can be conceptualised as having the 'potential' to become structured into and identify with probation discourses.

Technical discourse was less prevalent in records on black offenders, whose offending was more likely to be partially situated outside the official discourses which classified and framed explanations for offending and recommendations for disposal. It was not simply the case that white offenders were presented as being more amenable to the transformative process of the good subject, whereas black probationers were delineated within the discourse of the bad subject who refused to identify with the probation officer in an act of counter-identification. A more complex array of discontinuous theme selection served partially to remove the black offender outside a rehabilitative discourse more easily recognisable to probation officer and sentencer. The probation officer also constrained by social-work discourses appeared to move with uncertainty between the conventionality of doing 'something constructive' and an inability to express the phenomenon presented by the black offender within the discourse required by the criminal justice system. In the above instance previously described (p. 69) and quoted below, explanations for offending are framed to give an appearance of a humanistic social-work discourse. Gaps are created in the discourse that seriously limit the possibility of the defendant becoming a good subject. Thus although the black defendant was depressed, a word like boundary invoked an imaginary professional specificity:

> He threw a drain grid through a shop window on each occasion and stole watches and items of clothing from the displays. I gather that some of these goods were recovered. The defendant adds that they were items he neither wanted or needed, and can offer no explanation for what he says are spontaneous acts of folly.

This brief section of probation discourse suggests how:

> One is confronted with concepts that differ in structure and in the rules governing their use which ignore or exclude one another.
> (Foucault 1972: 37)

The themes introduced by the probation officer are dispersed throughout, are not organised in any progressive or deductive structure. Specific mention of the drain grid could serve to dramatise the offending act, while the recovery of the goods lessens the effect of the offence. The sentence that follows serves to reference the client's explanation outside probation discourse. The offender did not need the goods and therefore describes the act himself as a 'spontaneous act of folly'. The last part of the sentence leaves room for the possibility for the creation of a good subject since it includes the possibility that the offender has understood the nature of his own actions. The term 'spontaneous acts of folly' is framed somewhat unconvincingly within the discourse of the white professional welfare worker. In this section of the report, as Foucault has suggested, various 'strategic possibilities' are presented to the probation officer that permit the activation of 'incompatible themes' or, again, the establishment of 'the same theme in different groups of statement'.

FILLING GAPS AND EMPTY SPACE

Thematic dispersal in social-enquiry report presents the reader with an apparent series of gaps which are intertwined with one another, creating 'interplays of differences, distances, substitutions, transformations' (Foucault 1972: 37).

In seven white cases and two black cases the counselling relationships was seen as providing a 'space' for the offender to explore his relationships with people. All probation officers who used this term were asked in second interviews to define what they understood by space in the context of their work with that offender. Four different meanings were given for what was being attempted, while in three cases the probation officers were unable to define the term and expressed some surprise that they were being asked to do so.

Space for one probation officer was 'an obvious part of casework', although four meanings were given in relation to this concept. In one of the examples involving a black offender it emerged that the officer was referring to physical space, or the place in which an offender could come on a regular basis in order to discuss problems.

Second, also in a situation involving a black offender, space was created away from the 'daily grind of life' in order to consider feelings and relationships with other people. A third meaning can best be described as an ontological form of space which enabled 'offenders' to explore their own feelings in order to enhance the nature of their own existence in the social world. This was used in relation to white offenders and was expressed in the following manner by a probation officer:

> X has never understood his own position in the world, he can't understand why people react to him in the way that they do. Our talks together have given him the space to do this.

Space was used, in a fourth sense, to describe a punctuation mark in the counselling process in that the probation officer in the interview describes herself as 'Holding off to give him space to think about what we've spoken about'.

Numerous other examples of such linguistic practices abound in the research. The idea of 'working through problems', 'confronting offending behaviour', 'denial' and 'starting from where the client is' frequently occurs. The use of such terms suggests the presence of conventions governed by rules possibly unrecognisable to those who use them. Power can be seen to be operating in a number of directions. If the probation officer is successful in persuading the courts that a non-custodial 'disposal' is appropriate in a particular instance by utilising power through a professional discourse on behalf of a defendant, gestures of domination and submission are continued into the period of probation. Counter-strategies of subversion and evasion are in turn developed by the probationer. What appear to emerge are a number of frameworks within which practice is conceptualised, each with its own language, logic and set of meanings.

CLASSIFICATION AND FRAMING OF SOCIAL-WORK KNOWLEDGE

The notion that discourses have natural boundaries and constitute 'unlocated universes of meaning' is rejected by Rodger. He argues that discourses develop out of conflict with other challenging and competing discourses. Following Bernstein, Rodger argues that the most appropriate way of engaging in discourse analysis in the sphere of welfare is to study the classification and framing of knowledge in the social-work professional 'client relationship':

There is no single professional discourse dominating social work practice but rather a variety of 'negotiated' discourses emerging from particular localised encounters between individual social workers and their clients.

(Rodger 1991: 77)

The need for the development of emancipatory linguistic competence in social-work practice is developed by Rodger, who argues that a subjectless social work can lead to a world devoid of subjects. While agreeing with Rojek and Collins that post-structuralist thought reveals how power is mediated through social-work discourses, he is less convinced that the approach offers guidance for practice, if it:

Eliminates the political level of conflict and resistance which is always possible in professional-client relationships, and always involves acting knowledgeable subjects.

(Rodger 1991: 68)

While post-structuralism leads towards a 'metahistory of social work' and an 'excavation of the linguistic', Rodger argues that other sociological perspectives like ethnomethodological analysis can focus attention on the everyday life of social-work practice, the:

Taken for granted world of social interaction where distorted communication becomes solidified by the real material circumstances of poverty, class, and racism, and needs to be dissolved by the social worker if any assistance is to be offered to overcome immediate problems.

(Rodger 1991: 69)

Rodger combines an ethnomethodological form of analysis with a coded classificatory schema in an attempt to relate the archaeology of social-work knowledge to everyday processes. A code is defined by Dimbleby and Burton as a 'system of signs bounded by conventions', while the term convention is used to describe the:

Rules defining how signs are used within codes and how these signs are collectively understood.

(Dimbleby and Burton 1985: 204)

Bernstein uses the concept of code in his analysis of educational systems to specify two basic processes which govern boundary relationships between different spheres of knowledge. The *classification* of knowledge is strong where there is a degree of insulation between the contents of knowledge and the 'statuses of knowing'. This can be seen as strong in the teaching of 'pure' subjects like geography and history, but weak when called modern or general studies. The *framing* of knowledge is strong when teachers have the power to control learning, but weak when learning is controlled by pupils or students (Bernstein 1973).

In the collection code the contents of different knowledges stand in relation to each other, e.g. pure combinations of science or humanities at 'A' level. The integrated code favours a more flexible, open relationship between the contents of knowledges not found in collection codes. Collection codes are characterised by strong classification and framing of knowledge, whereas integrated codes are more likely to produce weak classification and framing of knowledge.

Rodger relates these concepts to social-work practice by substituting collection codes with correctional codes and integrated codes with appreciative codes. The appreciative stance in social work, Rodger argues, encourages social workers to acknowledge and understand an individual's qualities without seeking to challenge them. Instead:

> A correctional code tends to view problem populations as being in society but not of it, whereas an appreciative code views problem populations as the creation of society.
>
> (Rodger 1991: 72)

It has already been suggested that white probation officers tend to conceptualise black offenders within a correctional rather than an appreciative code. The way in which words are placed in relation to one another constitutes linguistic conventions which are seen in both written and verbal forms of communication. It would appear that in the discourse of the court an appreciative code can only be adopted when certain conventional requirements have been met: or, put more precisely, both probation officer and sentencer can make it appear that they have been met. As Rodger suggests this process of agreement is arrived at by:

> A variety of 'negotiated' discourses emerging from the particular, localised encounters.
>
> (Rodger 1991: 78)

The classification and framing of knowledge into the conventionality of technical language enables probation officers to reconstruct
paradox as coherence (Cousins 1978: 70). The code created by the
discourse will endorse a vocabulary of motive which is either
acceptable or unacceptable for the creation of client status.

One of the central concepts governing the selection of codes
is the notion of individual responsibility. If the probation officer
judges that the offender voluntarily committed the offence, then
conventionally a corrective code is adopted. If the behaviour
is attributed to some external force, e.g. sickness, addiction,
temporary aberration, effectively removing the voluntarism of
the offending, the appreciative code is more likely to be used.
Complex combinations of codes are employed randomly at times,
although in all reports one code can be said to be emphasised or
repeated. Of the 21 explanations of offending found in social-
enquiry reports submitted to the courts, 16 suggested that in
some way the offending was to varying degrees beyond the
control of the offender. Other explanations like irresponsibility,
instinctive criminality, anger and anti-authoritarianism suggested
that offending emanated from forms of individual pathology.
The offender had chosen to offend, in some cases 'frivolously'.
Such explanations were used almost exclusively to describe black
offending. Anger was frequently related to racist attacks and the
offender's feelings about racism, yet anger was emphasised as being
the cause of offending.

Racism is not a concept that is readily utilisable within the conventional systematicity of probation discourse. Figure 4.3 summarises
the line of argument which might be relevant to future analyses of
probation practice. The offender worthy of clientisation becomes a
victim of circumstance and is in the process of becoming a 'good'
subject. The discourse is referenced within the micro-domain. This
enables the probation officer to argue that the techniques at her/his
disposal are relevant in the task of rehabilitating the offender, thus
validating her/his professional position within the wider criminal
justice system. The offender then gains entry into the probation
system.

Negative connotators are often used to qualify and severely
affect the vocabulary of motive leading towards the offender being
presented as a threat. The defendant is enunciating a position which
could call into question the usefulness of the probation officer's
professional skills and values. The offender is also refusing to

identify with the discourse or, as in the case of many black offenders, adopting an alternative discourse. The offender can also be conceptualised in terms of becoming a threat to those who appear to identify with the discourse, e.g. probation officer and sentencer.

Black offenders who cite racism as a 'causal factor' in offending are more likely to be subjected to the correctional code and its associated discourses. It would seem, then, that when the probation officer is faced with an unconventional explanation like racism, a number of possible strategies can be employed. One often preferred option is to ignore racism in explaining offending to the courts. Alternatively, the probation officer may contextualise the explanation of racism given by the black offender within a correctional code, appreciative code or a combination of both. It is the code or code-emphasis that will to a significant degree determine the selection and distribution of themes within the explanation of offending and in consequence differentially affect what is signified to the sentencer.

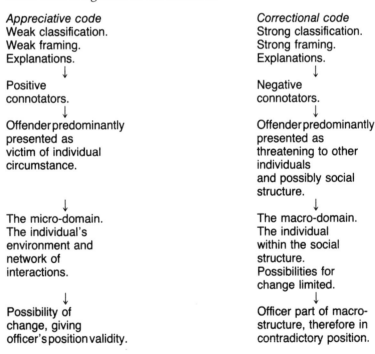

Appreciative code	*Correctional code*
Weak classification.	Strong classification.
Weak framing.	Strong framing.
Explanations.	Explanations.
↓	↓
Positive connotators.	Negative connotators.
↓	↓
Offender predominantly presented as victim of individual circumstance.	Offender predominantly presented as threatening to other individuals and possibly social structure.
↓	↓
The micro-domain. The individual's environment and network of interactions.	The macro-domain. The individual within the social structure. Possibilities for change limited.
↓	↓
Possibility of change, giving officer's position validity.	Officer part of macro-structure, therefore in contradictory position.

Figure 4.3 To show appreciative and correctional codes in probation practice

CONCLUSION

In order for probation officers to advance beyond the conventions of professional discourses, attention must be given to the ways in which the providers and recipients of the service assemble meanings through competing discourses. Language is fundamental to the work of probation officers, whose task it is to extract the 'truth' surrounding criminal behaviour from a number of sources including the defendant, other social workers, official records, reports, the medical profession and the police. From this variety of differing and competing discourses, an official explanation of offending is assembled and a 'treatment' plan produced, which will have legitimacy in court. The linguistic rules of engagement require the probation officer to collate and translate explanations of unlawful behaviour into codes recognisable to official judicial bodies. The deconstruction of official discourse could provide the beginnings of a process that penetrates dominant and discriminatory conventions. If attention is not directed to deconstructive analysis of the meanings that black people impute to their own behaviour, correctional codes will be structured into professional language:

It is crucial that the meaning of words as they are utilised by people in everyday contexts (first order constructs) is grasped when negotiating contracts or agreements. If the language of the professional discourse (second order constructs) is given priority by the social worker then communication is more likely to break down.

(Rodger 1991: 76)

Thus when black people attempt to describe their offending, the logic of racism must not be imposed or translated by probation officers but emerge from what Mills refers to as the 'vocabulary of motive' (Mills 1940, in Rodger 1991, p. 76).

Probation training is an obvious place for the 'vocabulary of motive' to be examined, yet it is not currently included in social-work curricula. In discussing the training of social workers, Pitts argued that social-work students should:

Equip themselves to navigate the space between the white powerful authority figure and the black young person whose only power lies in the ability to resist or confound our often incomprehensible overtures.

(Pitts 1984, quoted in Ely and Denney 1987: 190)

Competing official and unofficial discourses, even though they constitute two relatively autonomous sites of struggle, currently play no part in the training of probation officers. The social-enquiry reports prepared by probation students on placements during their training could provide vital analytical and assessment material. In constructing explanations of illegality for the courts, the probation officer must attempt to understand both the vocabulary of the offender and the construction of their own discourses.

Chapter 5

Racism, anti-racism and probation policy

The official policy position on race-related issues and the probation service is unequivocally expressed in a Home Office circular:

> The Home Office is wholly committed to the elimination of racial discrimination from all aspects of the work of the probation service, and to a policy of racial equality. There must be no racial discrimination of any kind, conscious or inadvertent.
>
> (Home Office 1988b)

This chapter examines the effects of Home Office and local policies on the development of probation practice with black people. After a brief historical discussion, the genesis of policies that have shaped the provision of services for black people at central and local level will be examined.

THE LEGISLATIVE BACKCLOTH

The wider trajectory of national 'race relations' policy provides a context for understanding policy formulation within the probation service. The circular that formulates the basis for policy in the area of race expresses an expectation that probation committees will promote a policy of equality of opportunity for employment and advancement in accordance with the Race Relations Act of 1976. Some of the contradictions inherent in the race-relations legislation are to some extent reflected in probation policy.

The 1948 Nationality Act ensured the right of colonial passport-holders as well as those holding passports issued by independent Commonwealth countries to enter the United Kingdom freely, to settle, find work and enjoy full 'political and social rights' (Radical

Statistics Group 1980). Such a policy reflected not only a postwar need for labour but also the American melting-pot ideology, whereby the 'dark strangers' would become assimilated into a flexible and tolerant society. The goal of assimilation continued through the 1960s. The prevailing view among policy-makers was that racial harmony depended on the elimination of cultural barriers. The 1962 Commonwealth Immigrants Act restricted the automatic right of Commonwealth citizens from entering Britain, creating a voucher system which was related to occupational skills. This legislation appears to have been based on the premise that racial tension, which had surfaced in some urban centres such as Notting Hill and Nottingham in the late 1950s, could be ameliorated by a thinning-out of the black population.

In 1966, Roy Jenkins changed the policy agenda from assimilation to integration when he condemned assimilation as a 'flattening process' and called for a strategy characterised by 'equal opportu-nity', 'cultural diversity', and an 'atmosphere of mutual tolerance' (Jenkins 1966). Legislation does not appear to have followed this pattern since the 1968 Commonwealth Immigrants Act withdrew the right of settlement of those who did not have a 'close connection' with the United Kingdom. In order to have a 'close connection', an individual had to be born in the United Kingdom or descended from parent or grandparent resident in the UK.

Controls on immigration became ever tighter with the creation of 'patrial' status in the 1971 immigration legislation which defined the right of entry to the United Kingdom in terms of birth, naturali-sation or citizenship of parents or grandparents. Non-patrials who had been granted permission and a work permit were admitted initially for a period of one year. The British Nationality Act 1981 was designed to 'clarify' the concept of British citizenship but in practice further tightened entry restrictions. A child born in the UK can only acquire citizenship if either parent is a British citizen or ordinarily resident in the UK. The definition of ordinarily resident is difficult to define and in any event is defined by an immigration officer and not a court.

Legislation designed to curb racism was introduced in 1965 and 1968. The current legislation contained in the 1976 Race Relations Act makes it an offence to publish or distribute written material or use language in any public place which is threat-ening or abusive to black people or is likely to incite racial hatred.

In the model race-issues policy statement for probation committees, the Home Office contextualise action with reference to this
contentious piece of legislation. It is widely acknowledged that
the Act has been ineffective in combating racial discrimination.
The Commission for Racial Equality argues that a new law should
improve the definition of indirect discrimination and improve the
procedures and remedies available in racial discrimination cases in
order that action can go wider than the individual case. Legal aid
could also be extended to discrimination cases, while an equal-
opportunity division could be created within the industrial-tribunal
system (CRE 1990).

Hepple has argued against a 'naïve instrumentalism' which sees
current legislation as having a specific purpose against which effectiveness can be measured. Critics of the Act, he argues, are wrong
to blame the legislation for the enduring reality of racism. Hepple
rejects the view that by giving the Act more teeth through the
imposition of deterrent sanctions that an impact on discrimination
could be made. Legislation should be seen as an instrument for the
negotiation of change and the creation of symbols around which
struggles for change can be organised. Legal concepts by definition
need to be specific and cannot individualise conflict between parties
(Hepple 1987).

PROBATION POLICY AND THE CULTURAL
MELTING POT

The police-court missionaries of the nineteenth century were
concerned with bringing individual redemption to recalcitrant
souls. The Probation of Offenders Act 1907 first gave magistrates
permission to appoint probation officers, but it was not until 1925
when the Criminal Justice Act created probation areas that the
beginning of the probation service as it exists today began to
develop.

Throughout the late 1930s and 1940s the probation service went
through a 'phase of diagnosis', with an emphasis on the quasi-sci-
entism of assessment and treatment of the individual (McWilliams
quoted in May 1991: 15). This provided the probation officer with
a professional status based on an ability to perform individualised
work with offenders. It is to this period that we must look for a
partial explanation of the beginnings of the techno-language presented
in Chapters 3 and 4. The focus of probation work was directed

away from the reclamation of souls towards the quasi-psychiatric assessment and treatment of inadequate personality traits which led to criminal behaviour.

The post Second World War recruitment of black people from the New Commonwealth and Pakistan by the British government does not appear to have influenced probation policy until the early 1980s. The late 1950s and early 1960s saw the numbers of probation officers increasing as duties expanded. The role of the probation service was extended to matrimonial proceedings in 1958. In 1966 the probation service took on the duties associated with the movement of 'after-care' from the Voluntary Prisoners Aid Association. In 1967 the Criminal Justice Act further extended the role of the probation officer to cover parole (May 1991).

The emphasis of integration over assimilation as a basis for government race-relations policy in the mid to late 1960s was contemporaneous with the development of 'therapeutic optimism' (Willis 1981) and a belief in what Raynor calls 'emancipation and enhanced possibilities' in the aspirations and goals of the probation service (Raynor 1985: 3). Such policy orientations do not appear to have extended to a detailed consideration of the emancipation of black people, despite the enduring reality of material poverty and racial discrimination in education, employment and housing endured by black people (Rex and Moore 1967, Smith 1977). One of the very few references made to black people in the 'probation literature' of the period can be found in an article by Wallcott in which references are made to 'overcrowded living conditions' and frequent disagreements within the black extended family. Other new influences like pornography are also identified as being causally related to black adolescent crime. Black people and black families in particular are conceptualised in deficit terms (Wallcot 1968).

May characterises the 1970s as the period of piecemeal diversification, with an emphasis on teamwork which was thought to provide a 'liberal ground' mediating 'radical left attacks' and the 'justice model' (May 1991: 35)

Until the early 1980s something approaching an avoidance strategy was taken by both probation managers and the Home Office in relation to policies necessary for the beginnings of an anti-racist probation practice. It was in 1976 that a study of Merseyside probation suggested that probation officers might be

making fewer non-custodial recommendations for black offenders
(Husband 1980).

In an apparently contradictory move by the Home Office,
Rastafarians were effectively denied the right to exist in the prison
establishments. In a Home Office circular it was stated that:

> It has been decided that Rastafarianism does not qualify as a
> religious denomination for the purposes of section 10 (5) of
> the Prison Act 1952 which requires a Governor to record on
> reception the religious denomination to which a prisoner declares
> himself to belong.
>
> (Home Office 1976: 1)

Although this unexplained regulation was subsequently revoked,
it indicates the insensitive and contradictory position taken by
the Home Office in the mid-1970s. Failure to recognise Rastafari
was guaranteed to create further resentment in a prison system
where black people were already over-represented. The 1976
circular made nonsense of the subsequent Home Office circular
which appeared in 1977. This called upon probation areas with
a significant black population to appoint an officer with special responsibilities for the development of appropriate services
for 'ethnic minorities'. The Home Office exhorted probation
officers to adopt a professional approach to the 'ethnic' dimension of their work. Any differential treatment of black people
by probation officers was based upon the inability of individuals to carry out cultural adaptation: a situation exacerbated by
a lack of information on the services that were available to
black people. Cultures were conceptualised in terms of coherent
self-sufficient systems that needed to be protected by policies.
Specialists with knowledge of differing cultures could resolve
cultural conflicts and misunderstandings (Home Office 1977).
What can be discerned from a number of official documents is
a preoccupation with the 'immigrant' who was conceptualised as
being deprived and lacking when measured against an imaginary
white standard of normality. It did not take a great conceptual
leap to link deprivation with 'ethnicity' to create deficit cultural
assumptions.

The Bristol disturbances of 1980 and the widespread unrest
in Brixton and other inner city areas which followed in 1981
emphasised the need for a policy that not only recognised the
existence of institutional racism within the probation service, but

contained practical policy-related suggestions that would create the framework for an anti-racist probation strategy.

MONITORING A PROBLEMATIC RESPONSE

Despite more protests and loss of life on the streets of London in 1985, the Home Office appeared unable to take decisive action in beginning to address racial discrimination in the probation service. Monitoring was the major response of the 1980s. The West Midlands Probation Service and the Commission for Racial Equality initiated the first major local study of probation work with black people in the West Midlands (see account of Taylor (1981) in Chapter 1). Like many of the early local studies mentioned in Chapter 1, Taylor's quantitative work helpfully described the inequalities in service delivery through a monitoring process, but it stopped short of any firm policy conclusions.

Monitoring can be seen as a device whereby an appearance of action to solve the 'problem' is created: a measure which is arguably more associated with crisis management than with challenging the underlying policies and practices which create the differential treatment of black people in the criminal justice system. It can be argued that the mere act of asking about 'ethnic origin' can be conceptualised as racist. Such questions can appear to make black people become defined as the problem, while the institutionalised arrangements in the criminal justice system which discriminate against them are not so defined. This argument is frequently countered by the need of policy-makers to form a quantitative basis to assess future policy requirements. If managers monitor, they can be accused of delaying tactics, while if they fail to monitor they may leave themselves open to the charge of ignoring the structured subordination of black people.

This dilemma is exemplified in a recent attempt at 'ethnic monitoring' carried out by the Home Office which consisted of a census of clients and probation staff. The classifications used by the Home Office which include white, black Caribbean, black African, black British, Indian, Pakistani, Bangladeshi, Chinese, others and not known, appear to seek the nationality of offenders and employees of the probation service. This approach is justified on the basis that data relating to different ethnic collectivities is required in order to understand the extent to which discrimination is experienced within different subgroups. Such an approach is regarded by NAPO as an unacceptable use of private information, effectively utilising categories of nationality to divert attention from the relationship between skin colour and discrimination within the criminal justice system. Monitoring, it is argued, should be more properly directed towards measuring the impact of anti-racist policies on probation practice and policies (NAPO 1991).

In a document published by the 'race forum' set up in the West Midlands service by the ethnic minority liaison advisory group in 1981, the complexity of this and other debates relating to monitoring in the probation service was discussed. The process of monitoring should go beyond a counting and categorising exercise and provide a method whereby probation officers can 'think before they write'. The forum called for monitoring to include analysis of references to:

Race, colour, creed, nationality, country of origin, or ethnic background.

Monitoring should also extend to 'value judgements', the 'projection of dominant white culture' stereotyping, 'identifying instances and recommendations of disparaging comments', and an examination of 'no clear recommendation against custody' (WMPS Race Forum 1984).[1]

A further concern related to the use of monitoring in probation is the purpose to which information will be used and the fear that information gathered by an organisation which is an integral part of the criminal justice system may eventually be utilised for surveillance purposes. A crucial determinant of the usefulness of a monitoring exercise lies in both its clarity of purpose and the sensitivity with which questions are posed. The design and rationale underlying any monitoring exercise has to be made clear from the outset in order to avoid the charge of tokenism.

POLICY INITIATIVES AFTER 1981

The inner-city disturbances in the early 1980s led to a series of policy statements which related more directly to the differential treatment of black people by probation officers. A report from the Central Council of Probation Committees (CCPC 1983) recommended a more proactive approach towards working with black people.

Ethnic liaison officers were thought to have been ineffective. The remedy to the 'problem' was couched in terms of more in-service training and pressure was applied to probation staff to attend. White applicants to the probation service expressing racist attitudes, it was argued, should be eliminated at an early stage. More black applicants for Home Office sponsorship should be encouraged, while the probation service, through such measures as the relocation of offices, should make themselves more accessible to black people. An imaginative but generalised community focus to probation work was advocated, which, it was argued, would make the probation service more relevant to black people.

A report by the Association of Chief Probation Officers suggested that the probation service should play a crucial mediating role between black people, the police and the courts: a suggestion which was a clear response to later inner-city disturbances (ACOP 1985).

Some probation officers working with black people in inner-city areas were suspicious of a more community-oriented policy for a number of reasons. First, there was an inability or unwillingness to change the way in which they worked (Carrington and Denney 1981). Other officers drew attention to the unintended consequences of community-oriented initiatives instigated by the Home Office. Writing in a collection of accounts of community-oriented probation, Scott emphasised that the move towards probation in the community suggested a greater surveillance role for the probation service (Scott *et al.* 1985).

The notion of the probation officer playing a role in the containment of black people reflects the development of a movement towards an element of punishment in the design of alternatives to custody. In a helpful commentary of change and conflict in probation-policy development, May describes the gradual emphasis of a justice-through-punishment model, which he argues leads to 'more of an element of control than care' (May 1991: 41). Populist discourse relating to the criminal justice system is based on the idea that 'violent crime is due to a softening of discipline, itself symptomatic of a breakdown of traditional values' (May 1991: 48).

It was the development and institutionalisation of a more punitive current of thought which to a large extent has made the community-oriented initiatives advocated pale into insignificance as the policy arena was prepared for the emergence of punishment in the community.

DIRECTIONS FORWARD

In the White Paper 'Crime, Justice and Protecting the Public' the Government sets out its proposals for changing the criminal justice system in England and Wales. Two central objectives in the White Paper could offer potential, the development of which could benefit black defendants. First, the attempt to create a more coherent framework for sentencing offers the potential for reducing racist sentencing practices. Second, the notion that imprisonment is generally a negative form of treatment is particularly important when discussing a group who are disproportionately represented in custody.

The underlying and guiding principles of the policy create considerable doubt as to whether the emancipatory potential within some of the ideas can be implemented in a way which could touch upon discrimination within probation practice.

The emphasis on 'just deserts', the principle whereby the offender is punished according to the gravity of the crime and not the criminal record, does not take any account of the existence of institutionalised racism. Other aspects of policy also appear to assume a form of social equality. Sentencing should express public abhorrence of the crime, protect the public, provide compensation for the victims and deter against reoffending. Before imposing a custodial sentence, the courts should be satisfied that the seriousness of the offence warrants custody, while providing reasons for arriving at the conclusion that custody is the most appropriate form of disposal. Probation should be combined with other penalties, including community service, and the courts should have powers to make curfew orders, possibly reinforced by electronic monitoring. Community penalties should be easier to enforce, with three clear stages of enforcement consisting of a warning, administrative action by the probation officer and recall to court.

Prisoners, it is argued, should spend at least half of their sentence in prison. The present position is that a minimum of a third of the sentence can be served in prison for sentences under one year before parole. More careful consideration should be given to prisoners serving sentences of over four years and remission for good behaviour would be abolished. If long-term prisoners are convicted of further imprisonable offences, the court may order the outstanding part of the prison term to be served in addition to any sentence for the new offence.

The Green Paper 'Supervision and Punishment in the Community' (Home Office 1990b) suggests a new approach to probation work, emphasising the basic requirement that the probation officer should respond to the wishes of the court, protect the public and gear their work towards crime prevention, while attempting to liaise whenever possible with the voluntary and private sectors. Probation officers are also required to 'produce results'. A reorganisation of the service is envisaged with 'stronger management' specialisms and economies of scale; an amalgamation of probation areas is suggested as a major development in this direction. Probation committees should operate more like 'boards of management', possibly with paid chairpersons some of whom could come from the private sector. An expanded role for a management centre is envisaged, with all funding being provided by central government. The movement towards a national service was combined with a belief that the probation service should be more closely involved in partnerships with voluntary organisations and profit-making organisations, with specific reference to the delivery of bail, supervision programmes, post-release work and civil work.

PUNISHMENT IN THE COMMUNITY

The notion of 'just deserts' as expressed in the White Paper reflects a populist call for firm punishment:

> Offenders should be punished according to the gravity of their crimes rather than their records. Those guilty of the most serious offences should go to prison for a long time.
>
> (Home Office 1990c: 3)

Sentencing, it is argued by the Home Office, should aim at expressing public abhorrence at the crime, punishing the offender, protecting the public, providing compensation for victims and reparation to the community, and deterring against reoffending. The development of individual responsibility for crime and the transformation of the offender into a useful citizen set the tone for the future of the criminal justice system. The Home Office appear to take the view that unlawful behaviour and racism are discrete and unrelated concepts. The combating of racism in the criminal justice system as a whole and in the probation service specifically is not an issue discussed in the White and Green Papers.

A third document, 'Partnership in Dealing with Offenders in the Community', was a more elaborated and explicit statement of the intention to create institutionalised links between the probation-service industry, commerce and charitable organisations (Home Office 1990c).

The National Association of Probation Officers welcomed the recognition of the need for a more coherent framework for sentencing and the greater use of community penalties, policies encapsulated within both documents. But NAPO considered them to be flawed (NAPO 1990a, 1990b). The overriding emphasis on 'just deserts' directs attention towards punishment, which unhelpfully takes precedence over crime prevention, reoffending, reform and rehabilitation. More specifically NAPO notes that Government plans for criminal justice 'conspicuously' failed to address 'race and gender issues' (NAPO 1990a). One reference is made to discriminatory processes in the criminal justice system, when in para 1.16 of the White Paper it is stated that:

> There must be no discrimination because of a defendant's race, nationality, standing in the community or any other reason.
> (Home Office 1990a: 16)

This acknowledgement is not developed into a discussion of measures that might be taken to combat racism. Neither does this reference acknowledge the extent to which racism permeates the probation service and the criminal justice system.

The implementation of ideas based on the political rhetoric of individual responsibility marks a fundamental shift from the probation officer representing the state's attempt to rehabilitate the offender, to the probation officer as the administrator of punishment in the community. Although the contents of the White and Green Papers have implications for black and white offenders, particular aspects of current government thinking have important ramifications for the development of anti-racist probation practice.

AN OVER-REPRESENTATION OF BLACK PEOPLE IN THE CRIMINAL JUSTICE SYSTEM

It has been argued in previous chapters that through the complexities of competing discourses in the criminal justice system, the probation service could be instrumental in perpetuating discriminatory sentencing patterns. Black people are proportionately more likely to be serving custodial sentences, which has resulted in an over-representation of black people in prison. In June 1989 according to Home Office statistics, 15.5 per cent of the male prison population and 24.2 per cent of women in prison were black. The over-representation of black people in the prison system can be seen most markedly when these percentage figures are compared to the 5.6 per cent of the general population not designated white in official 'ethnic' groupings (NACRO 1991a).

There are a number of possible explanations for the over-representation of black people in the criminal justice system. These range from at one extreme the conception of a growing black criminal class propagated by the new right and at the other, the criminalisation of black people by discriminatory practices within the criminal justice system (Gilroy 1987). Other new realist explanations of black crime emerged in the 1980s which fall between these two positions (Lea and Young 1984).

In a comprehensive analysis of race and criminal justice, Reiner argues that racism may be one factor among many which leads to discrimination in the criminal justice system. The current inadequacy of quantitative evidence leaves the question open as to the possible effects of other variables like age, gender and class. The most plausible suggestion for Reiner is that both racial discrimination and black offending patterns have played a significant part in the over-representation of black people in the criminal justice system, prison and parole (Reiner 1989).

Measures proposed to change arrangements for parole, if implemented, would have a differentially harsh effect on black people. The diminished likelihood of parole for prisoners serving longer sentences will further disadvantage black people, since 19.1 per cent of those sentenced to over four years are black (NACRO 1991a). Motivation to observe prison rules is further reduced if remission for good behaviour is abolished (Home Office 1990a).

When in prison, it is becoming increasingly clear that black people are more likely to encounter discrimination: they often find themselves at the bottom of complex prison pecking orders (Genders and Player 1989). In a recent study, 53 per cent of black and 14 per cent of white prison inmates felt they had been badly treated in prison (NACRO 1991b). Once in prison the over-representative black prison population are now less likely to gain remission and because of their position within prison society are more likely to come into conflict with other prisoners and prison officers. Such a policy, which makes increased resource demands on the prison system, could inflame the anger felt by black people in prison, some of whom feel a profound sense of injustice following court proceedings. The addition of days for misconduct will make further demands on prison resources and increase anger. Although this policy may satisfy an apparent desire to 'punish', it is difficult to understand how the proposals concerning parole can fail to inflame an already difficult situation in prisons. Although there is disagreement about the likely effects of the new measures on the prison population, NAPO claim that the prison population will increase significantly, eliminating the effects of any reduction in the use of custody resulting from other measures suggested in the White Paper (NAPO 1990a). The policy would also appear to run counter to the other expressed goal which is to create good citizens, since it is difficult to understand how serving longer sentences can prepare people for life in the community.

SURVEILLANCE AND THE COMMUNITY

The suggestion that probation officers should be involved in electronic monitoring to enforce tracking and curfews has provoked a fundamental debate about the role of the probation officer. The involvement of the probation service with techniques involving physical control represent the inclusion of physical restraint into the professional repertoire of the officer. This research suggests that some black people find existing non-coercive forms of probation work unacceptable and are less willing to become clientised than white defendants, many of whom see probation as an alternative to custody. Suspicion of white people with authority can make communication with black people difficult when officers utilise casework methods. In areas in which disproportionate numbers of black people are stopped by the police (Willis 1983; Policy Studies Institute 1983) the imposition of electronic monitoring in order to impose curfews could make the position of white probation officers completely untenable. The creation of a situation in which the probation work becomes identifiable with policing and the imposition of physical control could create unprecedented resentment among black people, much of which would be directed against the administrators of such a scheme. There are a number of fundamental principles at stake which make the idea of electronic surveillance unworkable. NAPO has suggested that in the trials that have taken place, courts have found it difficult to find circumstances in which tagging was necessary or useful. Problems were also experienced with defendants without settled housing, since landlords and landladies were reluctant to have premises modified to accommodate electronic surveillance equipment. NAPO views these developments as:

> An intrusive, passive and negative response to unacceptable behaviour. It fits ill with the White Paper's own principle that 'it is better to exercise self-control than have controls imposed upon them'.
>
> (NAPO 1990a: 23)

Electronic surveillance has also been opposed by the Association of Chief Probation Officers, the Police Federation, the Prison Officers Association, NACRO, the Howard League and the Prison Reform Trust (NACRO 1988). Such a coercive form of probation work could contribute to black resentment in delicately balanced inner-city communities, adding further complications to the development of work in the community.

This task is made all the more difficult by many of the measures contemplated in the new proposals for the criminal justice system. The possible development of national standards combined with the reduction of probation areas into larger, more cost-effective management structures could be counterproductive to imaginative work with black offenders. The result of this policy, if implemented, could be a probation service which is less receptive to local variations in need. Intimate and accurate knowledge of a locality is essential if the probation service is to respond to complex local needs. The creation of larger, possibly more bureaucratic probation-management structures could potentially slacken the pace at which a local service can responsively facilitate appropriate services for black people.

Other proposals offer the possibility of more relevant community interventions with black offenders. In the discussion document, 'Partnership in Dealing with Offenders in the Community', the development of partnerships between the independent sector and the statutory agencies is emphasised. The common thread running through the discussion is the wider involvement of the community in work with offenders to reduce crime (Home Office 1990c).

This book has suggested that white probation officers often fail to take account of existing projects which have been created and managed by black people. It can often be the case that probation officers could more properly be involved in resource provision for existing projects rather than instigators of new, less appropriate community projects. The emphasis on partnership with other organisations offers the potential for resources to be allocated to existing underfunded projects which are conceived and managed by black offenders. For this to be effective, a level of empowerment has to be accepted by resource providers in enabling black workers to develop projects in ways they consider appropriate.

COMBINING ORDERS AND BREACH PROCEEDINGS

The introduction of an order combining probation with a community-service order has particular implications for black people. It could lead to the imposition of community service or a 'high tariff' at an earlier stage in a defendant's life. A court dealing with a breach of such a combined order might feel that it had no alternative but to impose a custodial sentence in the event of two community alternatives being simultaneously ineffective. Such a measure could further add to the already disproportionate number of black people serving custodial sentences. The combined order could also place unrealistic demands on the subject, producing higher breach rates. The differential use of breach in relation to black people is a possibility that has received little if any research attention, especially when compared with studies of other areas of penal policy such as the sentencing of black people. Breach has been described by Fielding as the 'final sanction', marking as it does for many probation officers the negative signification of failure. In his study of 50 probation officers, Fielding found that three officers were unwilling to breach under any circumstance, while 21 would breach for extended failure to report or to keep in touch. Eight officers would breach for a failure to fulfil any condition of the probation order, including contracts made with the probation officer. Thirteen probation officers are reported as using breach in order to keep their caseloads neat. Fielding estimates that some 2 per cent of probation orders end in breach (Fielding 1984).

In the research described in this book, 4 per cent of the total sample, twice that found in Fielding's work, and 8 per cent of the black sample were breached. This was despite qualitative evidence that black people did not appear to miss appreciably more appointments than white offenders.

The empirical significance of such a quantitatively small sample is extremely limited, although this finding does raise an important question as to whether the breach proceeding is being applied differentially to black people. Any measure that increases the incidence of breach proceedings could also have a disproportionate impact on black probationers.

TOWARDS CORPORATE MANAGEMENT

The probation service is currently being led towards a corporate structure, adopting the ethos and management methods of a large national company. It is proposed that organisations dominated by the centre will probably become bigger, possibly more bureaucratic, and may ultimately be dominated by managers from the private sector. One of the methods by which this can be achieved is through the reduction and amalgamation of probation areas (Home Office 1990b). Although such a development may produce economies of scale in the short term, the creation of larger management structures could result in reduced morale among probation officers who feel unable to relate to larger management structures, while lessening the possibility of understanding the particular needs of black people in a locality. An inability of managements to be responsive to specific local needs could complicate the development of creative anti-racist practice in sensitive inner-city areas.

Any attempt to clarify the *modus operandi* of the probation service is a welcome development. Intervention that directly addresses offending behaviour and aims to reduce the possibility of further offending must be viewed as an improvement in the quality of the service offered. Unfortunately the issues involved are not as clear-cut as is suggested by the Home Office when they call on probation officers to justify the extra money being spent on the service through 'results'.

The measurement of the effects of developments in anti-racist probation practice are not easily quantifiable. We can illustrate this point with reference to the hypothetical example of a probation team developing a project designed to assist offenders in combating racism in the area of employment. Such a project might enable probationers and probation officers to explore jointly the ramifications and manifestations of racism in this crucial area of everyday life and may connect with the development of strategies for finding work. Practice of this kind may not immediately appear to address offending behaviour in the way intended by the Home Office. The value of such an approach lies in the potential for black people and probation officers collectively to gain confidence in tackling discriminatory behaviour. In a recent document entitled 'The Probation Service: Promoting Value for Money' it is argued that:

> While there is a striking variety of probation schemes in opera-
> tion involving much vision, creativity and imagination, these
> schemes must be evaluated, and their impact on offending behav-
> iour assessed. It is unsatisfactory that at present, considerable
> sums of money are spent with relatively little understanding of
> the effects achieved.
>
> (Home Office 1989: 2)

This Home Office statement appears to put imagination in a subsidiary position to cost-effectiveness. Probation officers should be encouraged to work with black people in a way which is both creative and efficient. It could well be the case that imaginative work creates longer-term effects on the offender, which are not measurable in the terms envisaged by the Home Office.

The proposed changes in the structure and financing of the probation service require new management systems which will be developed to comply with national standards of supervision and 'effectiveness'. Hitherto alien notions like 'quality control' could become a feature of day-to-day management if the new government proposals are fully implemented. Such measures will be essential components for survival in a competitive system in which the state-funded sector of probation could find itself competing for bids from private companies or trusts. The Home Office has already stated its intention to form partnerships possibly with independent companies or trusts in the delivery of some services, such as bail-support schemes (Home Office 1990c). The appropriateness of the private company being introduced into probation work is questionable. The implications for practice of such a demand/profit-led ethos within the probation service could further obfuscate the need for an effective anti-racist practice within the criminal justice system.

The cost-effectiveness of probation intervention as a method of addressing offending behaviour has been raised officially on a number of occasions during the service's history. Simple measurements of reconviction rates are fraught with dangers, since such crude quantitative measures fail to take account of crucial variables like population structures, e.g. age structures, previous criminal histories and the variable effectiveness of policing (Phillpotts and Lancucki 1979; Home Office 1988a). Racism and its causal relation to offending behaviour is another important factor which such quantitative studies fail to take into consideration. Some studies (Folkard *et al.* 1976; Raynor 1988) have shown that forms of probation work which have a clear, specific focus can assist the offender in social functioning.

The need for more offence-focused probation work cannot be over-emphasised in a book which has explored the relations between subjectivity, professional language and differential treatment. The pragmatic approach to probation work currently advocated by the Home Office rightly points to the need for the effects of probation work to be considered by probation officers.

LOCAL VARIANTS IN POLICY

In arguing against an over-centralisation of probation management and resource allocation, the need to adapt policy in accordance with local needs cannot be over-emphasised. In some geographical areas with long-established black communities, 'race-issues' policies developed by local probation services have produced disappointing results.

Divine describes some important research carried out in which four out of 17 black entrants to the local service failed to have their appointments confirmed at the end of the first year of employment. In these cases the supervising officers and managers involved in the decision-making process were white. Divine also found a divergence between black officers and management as to the purpose of probation work. Little guidance was given to black staff as to the framework of evaluation for confirmation. The service itself was seen as unwelcoming to black people, with managers displaying defensive and punitive attitudes towards black staff. Support for black staff was limited and the high expectations of black students was transformed into despondency by an oppressive organisational framework which appeared to marginalise black students. Divine comments:

The role of black staff in my opinion is qualitatively different to white staff in an agency. That indeed should be built into job descriptions and specifications. That does not mean to say that black people should only deal with black people. The agency therefore must be clear why it wishes to recruit black staff and convey clearly and directly to prospective black staff what tasks the agency envisages being performed by black staff. At present hidden agendas prevail.

(Divine 1991: 126)

The Home Office circular of 1988 stated that:

Work has already been carried out in some individual area probation services in developing an effective policy of equal opportunity for people of all races who come into contact with the probation services.

(Home Office 1988b: 1)

The word 'some' suggested the early stage of this area of policy development. One of the possible explanations for the preliminary state of policy formulation in the late 1980s is partially attributable to the view apparently taken by some officers at all levels within the service that policies designed to tackle racism were only necessary in black communities (Denney 1976). Relatively low numbers of black residents in some areas provided an erroneous justification for inactivity in this policy area. The Home Office now exhorts local probation management to apply 'energy' to race issues, requiring areas to provide a published statement of equal opportunities, detailed information and reports of racially discriminatory behaviour. It will be argued in the next chapter that more concrete proposals which affect daily probation practice are required if discriminatory practices are to be addressed.

FUTURE POLICY DEVELOPMENTS

Some of the most controversial measures contained in the punishment-in-the-community approach, including part privatisation and the creation of a national probation service, appear to have been modified or placed on ice, although the idea of a national framework of standards in most aspects of probation work will operate (Home Office 1991a). The overwhelming view that locally organised services should be retained has been partially recognised, although long-term funding arrangements for the service remain unclear. The Home Office intend to implement a tightly structured resource-planning mechanism with centrally determined sets of objectives which do not appear to address racism. Ideas contained in the new Criminal Justice Act of 1991[2] constitute an amalgam of concepts. Some of these have considerable credence in probation management and could have a profound effect upon the future of race-related policies in the probation service.

The introduction of the pre-sentence report for instance will provide the sentencer with the 'exclusive' responsibility for deciding on an appropriate sentence, while removing 'unrealistic' community disposals contained in current social-enquiry reports (Home Office 1991b). Although this limits the potential for racism in recommendations, it curtails the possibilities for incorporating an anti-racist perspective into the vital recommendations made in reports. Since other features of the pre-sentence report will remain unchanged, it will still be possible for officers to engage in forms of discriminatory subjectivity described in Chapters 1–4 of this book.

The history of probation policy in relation to black people creates a bewildering set of contradictions. It has been argued that current proposals for changing the criminal justice system in areas like parole and particular aspects of sentencing policy appear to increase the potential for discrimination in the criminal justice system. Other features of the policy, including the innovative appropriation of funds to projects managed by black people, with an increased emphasis on community penalties, could ultimately improve the quality of service. A concentration on improving the information made available to the courts could lead to less impressionistic and discriminatory social-enquiry reports. The enhancement of communication between the judiciary and the probation service could potentially allow probation officers to explain offending behaviour from the black defendant's perspective in less formal language than the social-enquiry report will allow. The default powers whereby action can be taken against a probation committee failing to comply with any statute or rule could be utilised centrally to ensure that anti-racist policies had some degree of effectiveness.

THE EXTERNALITY OF RACISM

Although strands of assimilationist and integrationist thinking have characterised official policies relating to the treatment of black people in the probation service, it would be oversimplistic to argue that policy has duplicated or even shadowed national legislative trends since the Second World War.

It has been suggested in this chapter that the development of probation policies in relation to race have been influenced by a complex of factors in addition to Home Office circulars and legislation. A number of themes do appear to link probation policy with the approach adopted by successive governments of both major parties. First, racism, a word notably absent from official discourse, is conceptualised in predominantly individualised and not institutionalised terms. The racist probation officer, like the recalcitrant probation client, can be trained into a non-racist form of practice. Black people and the site of their struggle appears to become manageable if referenced in such a way as to appear external to the criminal justice system. Second, as with the legislation, more stringent sanctions and controls which are likely to affect black people differentially are introduced, while simultaneously probation areas are called upon to implement equal-opportunities policies. Third, both national and probation policies appear to be managerialist in orientation, designed to contain potentially explosive situations while not addressing the underlying structural sources of discrimination.

The subordinate position occupied by black people in the criminal justice system remains for practical purposes unaddressed in the recent White and Green Papers. What emerges is a weak, incoherent and seemingly contradictory set of policies, which may lead black people to regard equal-opportunities statements made by local probation areas as little more than public-relations exercises. The responsibility for interpreting and utilising the potentially emancipatory elements of government policy in order to enhance probation practice for black people will fall not on those who frame and manage policy, but on officers who work daily with black people.

Chapter 6

Anti-racist directions in probation practice and training

In the previous literature, there has been a marked tendency to describe discrimination in probation practice. Researchers have taken the view that attention needed to be drawn to differential probation-service delivery before 'solutions' could be found. This final chapter examines some implications for practice which have emerged from discussions of research and policy.

RESISTANCE TO ANTI-RACIST TRAINING

The notion of race awareness popularised during the ascendancy of culturalism in the 1970s has now been transformed to the more active concept of anti-racist training. Awareness in itself is inadequate, since the overall aim of anti-racist training should be the active elimination of racism at the individual and institutional level. As Ahmed writes:

> Race awareness courses have been criticised for psychologising and individualising issues which are institutional in origin and require institutional interventions if they are to be tackled.
>
> (Ahmed 1991: 168)

Only four officers in this research reported having taken part in some form of race-related training. There did not appear to be any appreciable difference in the form of practice undertaken by the officers who had undergone training, although more specific research needs to be carried out to gauge the effects, if any, of anti-racist training on practice.

All four officers felt that they had gained valuable experience on the course, although the distinction between anti-racist training

(ART) and race-awareness training (RAT) was not made clear by officers interviewed. One officer spoke of feeling guilt at being white after the training. Another expressed a fear of the 'label' racist, realising that racism was wrong in practice and claiming that the atmosphere created in the workshop made it impossible to raise the question of how to tackle racism in his practice.

Two officers claimed that the entire issue had been 'overdone' since other equally important issues relating to social class, the position of women and ageism were also vitally important to practise and could produce differential service delivery. Officers claimed that the creation of 'guilt' in anti-racist training was counterproductive to developing their own practice. The major problem, as officers expressed it, emanated from a confusion as to what constituted the 'right' approach to working with black people.

Some workshops appeared to have left participants with the view that racism was biologically determined by skin colour. White people were by definition racist. Attention is focused on the individual pathological racist probation officer which could be seen as bearing a resemblance to the form of individualisation surrounding the pathologisation of black people in the criminal justice system.

Although anti-racist training is a vital part of the professional development of probation officers, the results of such training should be assessed and utilised. This aspect of anti-racist training is frequently ignored (Ahmed 1988).

In order to avoid such negative responses, anti-racist training and practice must be structured into every aspect of the probation officer's work. Anti-racist practice has to be conceptualised not merely as a set of ideas or guiding principles, but as a utilisable methodology running through all aspects of probation work. Specific exercises need to be developed which are grounded in daily activities like report-writing and assessments. The continuous self-monitoring of reports by teams is a process that enables officers to acknowledge the challenges they face in developing anti-racist practices. More elaborately, officers could be asked to produce reports on black and white people after observing mock interviews. The results could be compared in order to ascertain the basis on which information was included or excluded from reports. Such an exercise would also enable discussion of the way in which official explanations of offending were developed and presented to the courts.

RECORDING 'ACHIEVEMENT'

More recently probation officers have been required to be more disciplined and task-focused in their record-keeping. With the increasing emphasis on recording the 'results' of social-work intervention, the part c record has become far more uniform in nature and less like a short narrative. In many probation areas, records are no longer lengthy typed documents, but brief, hand-written records of contact. Such brevity could possibly reduce the scope for subjectivity in part c records.

Similarly, in part b records, the more structured form of record which makes it essential for the probation officer to list tasks prioritised and achieved might provide less opportunity for officers to express subjective opinions. On the other hand, such an approach may give officers the opportunity to be over-ambitious in setting goals and tasks which are unachievable. The ascendancy of the task-centred work model (Reid and Epstein 1977) in probation work during the 1980s cannot be considered in isolation from the Government's call for results and value for money. The effective officer, it is argued by some prominent writers on social-work practice, although well-versed in listening and counselling 'skills', should do something to assist the client to function in society as it exists and not indulge in outmoded Marxist dreams of revolution (Davies 1985).

Current probation-practice orthodoxy with its emphasis on action, although valuable in clarifying the purpose and effects of intervention, can create an over-reliance on the achievement of prioritised forms of functional behaviour within given time limits. The emphasis on the individual fails to recognise the importance of structural factors, particularly for black people. Such methods do not appear to include the task of combating racism. Discrimination in employment is apposite in considering the task-centred approach. Securing gainful employment is an intrinsic indicator of success, since at the point at which the order is made the subject agrees to live a good and industrious life. Such a task is severely hampered by racism, either overt or covert, and the possibility of building this into a contract between an officer and a black offender would seem to be almost impossible in an atmosphere in which probation officers appear to concentrate on individual deficit. It should be remembered that in any contract, the probation officer has more power than the probationer by virtue of his legal position. Such inequitable power relationships, however delicately hidden, are powerfully felt by a group who for generations have been subjected to the oppression of white domination.

Group-work was another popular method of work used by officers in this study which appeared to be of questionable relevance to black offenders. Groups appeared to be dominated by white officers and offenders, who were unable to appreciate the importance of racism in the lives of black people. Thus group-work, like the court-room situation, represented another sea of white faces within the criminal justice system.

A more appropriate model for practice might be an adaptation of the integrated approach which focuses on linking individuals with appropriate resource-providing systems. Such work would enable target systems to be identified within the process of change. In some of the examples of probation work given in this research, the Commission for Racial Equality and local black groups could be considered to be part of the client's system which could potentially be targeted by the probation worker to facilitate change (Pincus and Minahan 1973).

Attention must be directed at attempting to record precisely the effects of racism on the progress that black offenders make while in contact with the probation officer. The black person's own view of racism and its effects is an essential component of this process.

MONITORING

Reference to the problematic nature of monitoring has been made in Chapter 5. There are strong arguments for and against monitoring in probation work. Put crudely the argument for it is that without such an process the needs of black offenders cannot meaningfully be assessed, which inevitably results in the continuation of the colour-blind individualism described in this research. Thus systematic monitoring is seen to be necessary in order to understand the current needs of black people and the gaps in services. This has to be balanced against a fear felt by some probation officers and black people as to how such information will be used. Will it for instance be made available to the police?

This research appears to suggest that a more intensive process is required and should be instigated both locally and nationally. At the local level following the recommendation of the Central Council of Probation Committees there should be ethnic liaison officers in each area who are not, in the words of the committee's report, 'unobtrusive to the point of non-existence' (CCPC 1983: 1). At the local level a constant and rigorous process of monitoring could be undertaken. What this research clearly indicated, however, is that a counting exercise based on detailed 'ethnic' breakdowns does not constitute effective monitoring. At the national level, monitoring needs to be coordinated by an independent body in order to gain an overall view of the service being offered to black offenders.

BEYOND THE INDIVIDUALISATION OF PRACTICE

The call for probation practice which transcends black pathologis-ation extends over the last decade and a half. Quoting from a confidential Home Office report which drew attention to the differential treatment of black offenders in the probation service, Husband argued that black pathologisation sprang from probation officers' inability to adapt inappropriate, ethnocentric casework models to an essentially new situation in which second generation black people were challenging racism (Husband 1980).

The new agenda for an anti-racist practice has been clearly set out by Naik. Changes in the character, structure and operation of major institutions of larger society have to be accompanied by changes in practice:

> Local community-based institutions must be specifically con-ceived, designed and managed by members of the black com-munity. They must exert their energies to humanise the larger society by developing strong black alternatives to existing policies and institutions which will serve the needs of black people as a whole.
>
> (Naik 1991: 164)

Such themes have been taken up by other writers like Green (1987) and Whitehouse (1983) who have described innovative forms of community-oriented probation practice. One of the first probation-linked projects was the Handsworth Alternative Scheme in Birmingham. The aim of this project was to present the black offender to the courts in a more positive manner than had hitherto been the case, while concentrating practice efforts not only on the individual but on structural factors like education, employment and housing. Offenders were linked with training and housing projects, many of which had been developed by black people in the area.

Green describes the cultural centre in the West Midlands Probation Service, where the local service operates a community-centred form of work. Most of the staff and sessional workers are local black people who know the users of the centre at a personal level. The workers in the scheme tend to become involved at an earlier stage in the court procedure, not only as a result of a request from the court but on their own initiative. Green argues that one of the major advantages with this approach is that it recognises racism as a major contributing factor in black criminal behaviour. Black workers are able to understand the impact of racism on the lives of black people which makes the discourse between worker and users of the service significant and potentially helpful (Green 1987).

CULTURAL CAPITAL AND
RESISTANCE TO CHANGE

In Laketown the workings of a local black organisation, which in some respects resembled the cultural centre described above, were unknown to most of the officers who were interviewed. Mention was made by one officer that a black representative from the organisation was invited to speak at a staff meeting held by one of the teams involved in the research. Since the representative did not turn up, no further action was taken. What was remarkable about this research was the level of apparent disinterest which was shown in the potential benefits derived from working links with existing black groups.

The orientation by Green described above locates racism as being a central feature of probation intervention, thereby placing less emphasis on the conventions of individualist discourse which legitimate the white probation officer's conception of reality. Disappointingly, the initiative does not appear to have succeeded in increasing the use of probation orders at local level in the courts as it was intended to do (Green 1987). Such projects should be seen as forming integral parts of the local service and not methods whereby white officers can unload their responsibilities on to projects primarily designed for a 'racial' category. Some writers have suggested that black social workers are frequently used to fill a 'culture gap', creating the impression that something is being done about racism in service delivery (Stubbs 1985; Knowles 1990). The opposite and equally worrying tendency is for officers to underuse projects run by black people. Green reports that some officers have shown a reluctance in referring offenders to black-led schemes, many referrals being generated by representatives of the project (Green 1987).

A further practical problem stems from the fact that work of this kind tends to be funded on a temporary basis by staff who have little security and consequently move on to other more permanent posts. Such is the funding priority given to practice which addresses racism.

POWER COMMUNITY AND CHANGE – THE ROLE OF THE WHITE ANTI-RACIST PROBATION OFFICER

Projects that move racism into the foreground of probation work inevitably raise the question of how white probation officers can best make a contribution to the development of anti-racist practice. Knowles makes the important point that anti-racist struggles 'should be organised around issues and not qualifications for membership'. Anyone who is committed to challenging racism, black or white, can challenge racism and ensure that their own practice does not perpetuate discriminatory practices (Knowles 1990).

Husband has pointed to the paternalism implicit in white anti-racism which starts from a sympathy with the black person as victim. White anti-racism, he argues:

> Must surely be informed by each person's experience of oppression, and of being oppressive, in relation to those ideologies and forces constructed through class, age, gender or sexual preference.
>
> (Husband 1991: 68)

Recognising and working to change oppressive power relations is a necessary starting point for probation work which confronts the ramifications of racism.

If practices that challenge black pathologisation are to move beyond the margins of probation work, officers and management must be prepared to relinquish some of their power which will ultimately facilitate the black management of projects. Resource allocation and negotiating skills must be developed in order to enable black people to lead in developing services which are appropriate to the black community.

AUTONOMOUS INNOVATION

Such terms as separatist appear to be reserved for projects in which oppressed groups are attempting to work innovatively. For many years the probation service and judiciary were an all-white enclave and even now they are almost totally dominated by white people. Such features of the criminal justice system are never regarded as separatist. As Francis points out, there are many institutions whose clients are white which are not regarded as separatist. Since such community-oriented projects are granted such a small fraction of the total probation budget, a space has to be created for the development of new practices. A more appropriate word for such innovative developments is autonomous (Francis 1991).

In calling for a complete restructuring of the 'social-work system' Naik argues that:

> White control has been the most pervasive manifestation of racism in the system, the source of its greatest dysfunctions, and the most effective barrier to change.
>
> (Naik 1991: 161)

Official probation-service representatives on management committees of black projects might see themselves as representing the funding organisations, but could be perceived by the black workers who run the projects as reflecting, in Naik's words, 'white power'. In many instances the white social worker will be required to abandon white-oriented notions of social-work skills and assist in developing appropriate social-work facilities for black people. This could result in the probation officer utilising the power attached to being white, initially as a 'broker' in the allocation of resources for projects conceived and managed by black people. Officers and probation students must develop capacities to work within or to create organisational arrangements whereby black people can gain from available resources and utilise services not exclusively provided by the probation service. Such services may be created or maintained in partnership with established black groups in the community. Skills in qualitative and quantitative research are given scant attention on most social-work qualifying courses. Such activities are essential in understanding the resource needs of black people in the communities. The probation worker must demonstrate that she/he can negotiate with black-led organisations, white officialdom, probation management and the Home Office. Although there are problems involved with the efforts that have already been made to develop innovative forms of probation practice for black people, the essential advantages of such work can be seen in the beginnings of a willingness on the part of the probation service to recognise the reality of the black experience. The existence of projects that look further than individualised Eurocentric explanations of black offending need to be developed urgently if probation is to have relevance to black people.

FUTURE DEVELOPEMENTS IN PRACTICE

Although these efforts are important, a need for other forms of innovative practice are indicated by this research. Broadly this can be described in terms of including what has previously been referred to as the black offender's construction of reality into the routinised day-to-day work of the probation officer. Anti-racist practice, as Husband has argued, requires a conceptual location of the 'client' in their:

> Class, gender, and community context and explicitly acknowledging politics which have defined these statuses in predominantly 'race' terms.
>
> (Husband 1991: 65)

Thus the struggles against racism that many black people face in their daily lives should be recognised as legitimate within official documents such as pre-sentence reports and in all interactions with black people. The recognition of this reality partly removes the powerless and demeaning status of the client 'in need' and potentially offers a method by which the probation officer can have some measure of credibility with the black offender. This is essential for practice to have meaning to black offenders. The black person's right to a view of offending situated within the enduring day-to-day reality of racism must be recognised by the probation service in order to incorporate black reality.

A starting point for this process would be a reassessment of the presentation of offending in the pre-sentence report to sentencers. Racism can partly or wholly create responses within black people that lead them to situations in which they break the law. Thus the centrality of racism as a concept and a causal factor in offending must be acknowledged and explained to sentencers in reports when relevant.

Every possible opportunity must be taken to enable magistrates to have a broader understanding of the factors that influence black crime. This would require not just a shift in style but a reappraisal of the purpose of the social-enquiry report. In restructuring the way in which reports are written it is useful to refer to the seminal work of Bottoms and McWilliams (1979). In their 'non-treatment paradigm' they argue for a redirection of the probation service in the light of the collapse of the treatment model and suggest four aims for the probation service. These are: the provision of appropriate help for the offender; the statutory supervision of offenders; diverting appropriate offenders from custodial sentences; and the reduction of crime. They argue for a reconceptualisation of work involved with the writing of reports. Probation officers should move away from the language of implied moral judgements and develop practices that simultaneously aim to present the appropriate information to the courts while helping offenders develop strategies to prevent imprisonment.

Although this broad approach has applications to all offenders, it is of particular relevance to black people. There must be a clear sustained effort to remove Eurocentric judgements from all reports. The findings of this research reflect the lack of attention given to this area of practice on professional courses. Irrelevant subjectivity is so widespread that it needs to form the basis for any monitoring process. Such an approach must also concentrate on utilising information which is of direct relevance to the offence and which questions the use of more routinely included information, such as on school attendance or the probation officer's impression of the quality of familial relationships. It must also exclude accounts of families which connote stereotypical images of violent black parents. It would, however, allow the inclusion of other material which was not present in any of the reports examined in this research. This would include local unemployment rates, housing problems and other factors which differentially affect black people.

In advocating greater specificity in the writing of reports, we are not arguing for a complete exclusion of factors that relate to the offender's family or background. When mentioned, such material should be directly relatable to the offence in a way that incorporates the offender's view. It cannot be good probation practice to speculate in a quasi-scientific and uninformed manner on a black person's relationship with peers or family. Neither can it be good practice to fail to recognise the all-pervasive nature of racism and discrimination as phenomena which affect the lives of black people.

Morris and Giller have argued that the 'free-floating catalogue of pathology' found in many reports on offenders leads to the danger of the person being sentenced twice: once on the basis of the offence and once on the basis of his or her pathological problem and potential for future deviance (Morris and Giller 1987: 218. It is being argued here that black people might even be sentenced three times since they suffer the added burden of what has been referred to in this research as the negative connotations of the unconventional explanation. Black women carry the added load of sexist explanations which were also evident in this research.

COMMUNICATION WITH THE SENTENCER

The evidence relating to sentencing behaviour is complex and at times contradictory. While some studies find differences in sentencing which work to the detriment of black people (Stevens and Willis 1979; Walker 1988), other studies show no significant differences in the use of custodial sentences (McConville and Baldwin 1982; Moxon 1988). The use of differing statistical techniques and other factors add to the complexity of analysing sentencing practices in relation to black people (Mair 1986; Reiner 1989). While acknowledging all the difficulties in drawing firm conclusions from the evidence on sentencing, Hudson has argued that where offences are similar, Afro-Caribbeans are receiving custody and harsher alternatives to custody with fewer previous convictions than whites. Afro-Caribbeans have a shorter sentencing tariff and are less likely to receive non-custodial sentences (Hudson 1989). Probation practice forms only one part of the process that appears to discriminate against black people in the court-room.

Some officers in this study were reluctant to adopt a new style of report-writing that did not include moral judgements, innuendo and quasi-scientific conjecture, since they thought that such a style was expected by sentencers.

A number of possible ways of tackling this problem have been envisaged. Pinder, for instance, has suggested that a verbal account of offending given in the form of evidence in court might provide a less formal and stilted explanation of offending for black offenders (Pinder 1984). No evidence exists to support this view: if anything, the opposite applies, with Powell suggesting that some probation officers play an almost ritualistic part in the court process (Powell 1985).

The Home Office has recently endorsed the enhancement of probation liaison committees and magistrates court and called for more opportunities for the probation service to increase contact with the judiciary (Home Office 1991a). The probation officer can utilise formal and informal contacts with magistrates and judges to explain changes in practice and report-writing. This could also include meetings with sentencers and the production of explanatory literature for the consumption of sentencers by the probation ser-vice. Probation officers attempt to create opportunities for dialogue between sentencers and those who have been sentenced in order that black people can clarify the position they take in court. This is particularly important when considering Moxon's findings that black people in the Crown Court were more likely to contest their innocence than white defendants. This resulted in fewer reports being prepared on black people, with less likelihood of probation orders being made (Moxon 1988). This finding could indicate that black people are more likely to translate their perceptions of injustice into action despite the increased likelihood of a custodial sentence. The probation officer can play an imperative role in drawing attention to such features of the sentencing process.

Research needs to be done not just in the area of differential sentencing practices, but on the effects on sentencing of words used by probation officers in social-enquiry reports and verbal accounts of offending behaviour given in court: an aspect that was not included in this research.

CULTURAL CAPITAL – THE IRRELEVANCE OF SOCIAL-WORK THEORY

Theory was referred to in a wide-ranging manner. References were made to notions like casework and family therapy, although the nature of these forms of social-work theory were not made clear, despite the opportunities given to officers to do this in interview.

An overwhelming conclusion was that the form of work under-taken by the probation officer appeared to be led more by institu-tional demands than reference to theory or the expressed needs of

the offender. Such a demand-led service can emphasise the requirements of the system in which officers operate over the welfare of
the offender. The individualised and frequently unplanned nature of
much of the work examined in this research points to the delivery of
services on an *ad hoc*, reactive basis. Probation officers were 'trying
to get through the day', as one officer put it, having little time to
plan future interventions or reflect upon some of the judgements
already made.

This has clear consequences for both white and black offenders,
although the effects on black offenders were more serious. The
overwhelming emphasis on the 'individual' was structured into the
daily routine and requirements of the probation task, as were the
Eurocentric assumptions about the primacy of the nuclear family.
Considerable time was spent keeping often copious part c and b
records which were recorded into a dictaphone and typed by a
secretary. It was often difficult to see any relevance to the offence
in these records, many of which lacked reference to assessment, the
process of social work or the evaluation of work undertaken.

Some attempts were made at the first two processes, while there
was a notable absence of the third, i.e. evaluation. If probation
officers are to have an opportunity of understanding the effects
of their work, a serious effort must be made to assess the effects
of their intervention. It is only when this process of evaluation is
taken seriously by probation officers that discrimination in service
delivery can be tackled.

The relevance of theory which is forgotten, or thought to be of
limited value in daily probation practice, is raised by the findings
of this research. Theoretical ideas when mentioned were, as has
been suggested earlier, vague and ill-formulated. The officially
sanctioned method was task-centred casework, although on the
rare occasions when officers were attempting to agree specific tasks
with offenders over measured timescales, the tasks themselves were
unclear or too ambitious, as were methods selected for achieving
tasks. A cursory reading of the task-centred literature, a method
most frequently identified by officers, emphasises the importance
of clearly stating these two aspects of practice at the early stage of
the intervention (Reid and Epstein 1977). Effort has to be made
to enable theory to be a continuing part of the probation officer's
working life, if free-ranging subjectivity is to be avoided within
daily practice. Ahmed has argued forcefully that theory should
permeate social-work education and practice. Anti-racist materials

are available, written from a black perspective, which recognise relationships between race, class and gender. Such work tends to be found in journals unfamiliar to the white-dominated social-work education establishment (Ahmed 1991).

In Chapter 4 of this book a case was made for the beginnings of new theoretical departures that could enable probation officers to gain some understanding of the connotative value of the words used in explaining offending to the courts. This should be taught with reference to comparative case material on black and white offenders. Such a theoretical base could be used in service training, in the monitoring of pre-sentence reports and for teaching purposes on qualifying courses.

THE RECRUITMENT OF
BLACK PROBATION OFFICERS

In the Laketown probation service there was one black probation officer in employment when the research was carried out. Of the 6,651 basic grade probation officers employed nationally, only 127 are black. Only eight of the 900 senior probation officers are black and only two black officers occupy posts at the level of assistant chief probation officer (NAPO 1989).

The employment of black social workers as an anti-racist strategy, as has already been mentioned, has been criticised by a number of black writers. Gilroy warns that black social workers should not be drawn into managerialism which distances them from those who suffer the effects of racism. Neither should black workers be used to fill the 'cultural' gap that white probation officers are unable to fill (Gilroy 1987).

Even though black probation officers may not share the class position as black people on probation or in custody, if the forms of differential service seen in this research are to be avoided a major black influence is needed within the service. This will require changes within the recruitment processes which currently reflect a white-dominated service. Thus in identifying courses as being eligible for Home Office sponsored students, it might be stipulated that places be reserved for black students. This would require courses actively to recruit black students from existing access courses and white-dominated postgraduate courses could be compelled to make provision for black students. This condition should not be a matter of choice to individual programme-providers, but should be made a condition of acceptance of a Dip. SW programme by CCETSW.

A closer relationship between academic institutions and probation managers with responsibility for the development of anti-racist programmes officers would be required. Special efforts must also be made by local services to recruit black ancillary or volunteer workers who might be suitable for training. Positive efforts must be made to monitor recruitment and promotion within the probation service nationally in order to ensure that black people can reach positions in which they can facilitate change. Career opportunities within the probation service should therefore be advertised in the black press.

QUALIFYING TRAINING

Much of this book has been related to the development of training in probation work. Different approaches to practice require changes to be made in the structure and development of qualifying training for probation officers.

Hitherto, as has been suggested, a conspiracy of silence has existed in relation to the development of anti-racist practice in probation-qualifying training. An over-reliance on concepts suggesting a lineal normal form of development against which individuals can be measured has enabled social-work educators to remain incognisant of the need to develop anti-racist curricula and practices.

Courses have been able to claim impeccable anti-racist credentials on CCETSW validation visits, while still rooting teaching in the quasi-psychologism that dominated many of the social-enquiry reports quoted in this research. It is at the level of training that the roots of institutional racism in the probation service are laid. Probation officers learn the professional conventions which differentially affect black people in the criminal justice system while undergoing training.

Language issues and skills relating to the development of work with black people in the community have already been discussed. Students should also be provided with a basic appreciation of the legal background and requirements of the probation service. The ramifications of racism should be examined in relation to penal policy, rights and procedures under the race-relations legislation and aspects of criminology. Knowledge relating to the nature and ramifications of racism in the British social formation, interactive issues, e.g. family and naming systems, racist practices within the criminal justice system and the probation service must also be addressed. Students should be enabled to understand their own racism and its relationship to practice. Anti-racist training needs to be developed throughout the course in order to utilise practice experience. The 'buying in' of anti-racist teaching can serve to transform anti-racism into a separate 'thing' which is not part of the training course, shifting the responsibility for anti-racist training to 'specialists'. College-based staff must be fully committed to anti-racist teaching. The one- or two-day anti-racist workshop should therefore be seen as a starting point and not as an end in itself.

Lecturers (including staff brought in to teach in law, psychology or social policy) should explain to students how anti-racism is structured into their teaching. Social-work courses are frequently overloaded, with material reflecting attempts to cover vast amounts of material in too short a time. The result is often a bewildering amount of required reading, much of which this research indicates is ignored after training. Reading lists are unrealistically long and multiple copies of texts are rarely available at a time required by the students covering the same topic simultaneously. The assessed essay questions are often seen as being an almost ritualistic adjunct to the reading list. Through this minefield the student tries to navigate a course in an attempt to satisfy examiners.

A possible solution to these problems would be the requirement that each teacher prepare a module/component containing selected extracts from social-work theory and research material, with assessed essay questions or assessable exercises. Each student could be given a collection of materials for each component at the beginning of the course which would include anti-racist elements, collectively designed by teachers on the course. This would help ensure that students read essential materials required for the course in a way that integrated anti-racist perspectives.

The conspiracy of silence also extends to practice teachers who can still be selected out of a need to place the student. The student who experiences racist practices on placement may also be afraid to express anxieties for fear of being pathologised and 'failed'. CCETSW, with its power as a validating body, could play a key role in this area by providing in the last resort the protection required for students to expose racist practices on training courses and on placements. This will require CCETSW to have a higher profile on courses and open channels of communication for students. In the experience of the author, CCETSW is a somewhat remote and mysterious body to students.

Qualifying courses must indicate the way forward in their own practices by carefully monitoring teaching. Courses should prevent the burden of 'race expert' falling on black students by enabling all students to raise issues relating to oppression. Probation students, whenever possible, should undertake a placement in the criminal justice system which enables work with black people to be experienced. How this facility is provided by courses located in areas some distance from centres of black population when placements are at a premium needs to be addressed by course-providers, CCETSW and the Home Office.

Assessment should be an active process directly relatable to practice. Although the teaching of basic theoretical concepts is necessary on probation-training courses, it is insufficient for assessment to be based on a false distinction between the exposition of 'theory' in an essay or a three-hour unseen examination paper and the experience of practice. Assessment must be an integral feature of the practice running through the probation-training course. Opportunities should be created whenever possible for the products of placements to be used for the process of assessment and skill-development. Assessment could be focused more upon the production of work from simulated exercises, the analysis of part c recordings, assessments, plans for intervention and evaluations of practice. Ideas from sociology, psychology, social policy and social-work theory could be utilised in the analysis of practice. The ability of the student to focus on the effects of racism and strategies for combating racism could be targeted on particular probation tasks. The most obvious example of a product, as was suggested in Chapter 4, would be a pre-sentence report which could be used in skill-based components of the course. Other products could include video or sound cassette recordings of work with black offenders.

An alternative and possibly less attractive assessment model would be a separate compulsory assessed essay, an unseen written examination, or a series of objective multiple-choice examinations which addressed aspects of essential core knowledge, relevant to understanding the ramifications of racism in the criminal justice system. There is little evidence that such an approach tests the ability to apply core knowledge to practice.

Programme-providers should ensure that both the practice teacher and the social-work student address questions related to racism in probation practice on placement. The capacities developed during placement in relation to the assessment and evaluation of work with black offenders should be considered in full in the final report. Failure to consider the effects of racism in descriptions of work undertaken, as is currently frequently the case, is no longer acceptable. A practice teacher who is reluctant or incapable of addressing racism in the criminal justice system should not be approached by programme-providers. This requires that practice teachers also undergo anti-racist training that is not confined to a one- or two-day workshop.

At the end of the course the student would be asked to produce not a series of unconnected book-dominated essays, but a collection of materials gathered in a portfolio that developmentally represent various aspects of probation practice. Such a collection of materials would form the basis of the assessment, providing documented evidence of the student's ability to address and combat the contradictions created by racism. It could also be used as a resource in practice during the student's pre-confirmation year.

POSITIVE DIRECTIONS FOR THE PROBATION SERVICE

Dominelli has argued that individual workers can contribute to organisational change by breaking the 'conspiracy of silence' and speaking out against racism in their organisation (Dominelli 1988). Probation officers in this study had no structures through which they could challenge racism in their daily working lives, even if they had been so inclined. One of the most important points to emerge from this research was the lack of any coherent local policy in relation to the treatment by the probation service of black offenders. Despite the accumulating evidence indicating that black offenders are discriminated against in this area of social work, it would seem that the probation service has had sufficient time since Husband's initial work in 1976 to formulate policies which would make the service offered relevant to black people.

De la Motta reports that in the Nottingham area, the Association of Black Probation Officers, frustrated by the absence of a formulated national or local policy or policy statement, have considered the possibility of non-cooperation with management as the only way of expressing their anger (De la Motta 1984).

Implementation of any of the measures mentioned above is dependent on probation management understanding the importance of the discriminatory effect of current probation practices on black people. The Association of Black Social Workers and Allied Professionals produced a document in 1983 which suggested a list of four aims for practice in a multi-racial society with special reference to black families (ABSWAP 1983).

The findings of this research suggest that these aims could be adapted to probation practice. Probation officers, wherever possible, should strive to enhance and not deny the black identity of an offender. This will require knowledge of the objective position of black people in the social formation and more contact, both formal and informal, with black people. It will also require a clearer commitment on the part of CCETSW, qualifying courses, local probation management and the Home Office to provide suitable forms of qualifying and in-service training in order to achieve this end. The officer's attention must be directed towards the elimination of the racism that attempts to dehumanise and subjugate black people.

It is hoped that this book will make a small contribution to the recognition of the potential strength, diversity and challenge that black people offer to the workings not only of the probation service but to the wider communities in which they live. Until probation officers recognise the part that black people can play in nurturing new ideas within the probation service, they will simply be denying an enriching challenge and falling back on familiar but irrelevant practices.

Appendix

DESIGNING RESEARCH INTO
PROBATION PRACTICE WITH BLACK PEOPLE

Ethnography has formed an important part of this study which makes it necessary to clarify the concept. Hammersley and Atkinson usefully describe ethnography as:

> Simply one social research method albeit an unusual one, drawing as it does on a wide range of sources of information. The ethnographer participates overtly or covertly in people's daily lives for an extended period of time, watching what happens, listening to what is said, asking questions, in fact collecting whatever data is available to throw light on the issue with which he or she is concerned.
>
> (Hammersley and Atkinson 1983: 2)

Such a research approach enabled the researcher to explore the complexities of the social actor's definition of situations in a way that could not be measured in any positivistic sense. The fieldwork was undertaken over a six-month period in 1987. The researcher spent a total of 12 working weeks in the probation area, observing court-room procedures, team meetings and group interactions with offenders and in conversations with probation officers.

The selection of probation officers

Thirteen white probation officers took part in the study. In addition, one senior probation officer wished to make general comments about the issues connected with race and probation practice, while not wishing to comment on particular references to case material.

He argued that his current position precluded the possibility of constant contact with specific clients. White probation officers were selected for research, since the study was specifically focused on the official signification of 'race' in probation discourse. Much of the material analysed is drawn from the expressed views, reports and records of white probation officers. Non-participant observation in court and group interactions provided valuable research material, although the views of black people were often those reported or quoted by probation officers. A valid criticism of data collected in this way is that it provides a partial view of the phenomenon being examined. The findings of this research point to the urgent need for further research that concentrates more specifically on the way in which probation is experienced by black people.

Probation officers participating in the study were basic grade who had both black and white offenders on their caseloads. Seven of the officers were women, of whom two were non-graduates. Of the six men, four were graduates. The officers' periods of experience in the service ranged from one to 17 years. The officers who participated in the study also came from a wide variety of previous occupational backgrounds including military service, engineering, teaching, nursing, sales and publishing. All respondents had daily contact with black and white offenders. The group was largely self-selecting, given the size of the Laketown service and the relatively small number of black offenders. The probation officers who participated in the study were members of three teams situated in or near central Laketown.

The selection of clients

Research material was gathered on 50 offenders, 25 black and 25 white, all of whom were selected by officers. The officers also gained permission for materials relating to them to be examined anonymously by the researcher.

In order to gain a comparative quality to the research, an attempt was made to encourage probation officers to select clients who had a similar experience of the probation service, in that they had reached similar points in the tariff system and spent similar periods in custodial institutions. Probation officers were also asked to select black and white offenders who had committed similar offences. This was achieved to a reasonable degree through a simple process of pairing. Probation officers selected black offenders meeting the above criteria and then attempted to match them with other white offenders on their own caseloads. This resulted in a sample, 78 per cent of whom were between the ages of 18 and 25.

Probation officers were asked as far as possible to select offenders who had committed offences falling into the following categories:

a) The most common forms of crime against property, e.g. burglary, theft, criminal damage, going equipped for crime.
b) Offences against the person (those of a less serious nature).
c) Offences involving drug use.

Emphasis was placed on the forms of offending which occupy the major part of the probation officer's working time.

Gender

Although probation officers were asked to select offenders of both sexes, a greater proportion of male offenders were selected: 40 male offenders compared with 10 female offenders.

The research procedure

After negotiations with the Assistant Chief Probation Officer in Laketown, it was agreed that the researcher should attend team meetings in order to explain the research concern and methods. This was a useful exercise since the onus was on the researcher to convince the probation officers involved of the usefulness of the work. Having gained the agreement in principle within a public arena – the team meetings – full cooperation was gained collectively at a very early part of the research.

A small pilot study was undertaken with a view to testing the research instruments in the following sequence:

1 In-depth interview.
2 Transcription of in-depth interview.
3 Copy of transcription sent to probation officer for comments.
4 Analysis of social-enquiry reports and records.
5 Second interview with probation officer.
6 Comments from probation officers in team discussion with researcher.

A research project involving similar procedural sequencing had been successfully utilised in Pinder's study of probation practice with black people (Pinder 1984). It was thought essential to include material deriving from reports, records and interviews in order to gain a triangulated view of the research problem. Hammersley and Atkinson have argued that the multifaceted character of ethnography provides the:

> Basis for triangulation in which data of different kinds can be systematically compared.
>
> (Hammersley and Atkinson 1983: 24)

In-depth interviewing

The main difference between the way in which ethnographers and survey-interviewers ask questions is not, as is sometimes suggested, that one form of interviewing is structured and the other is unstructured. All interviews are structured by both the researcher and the informant. The important distinction is between 'standardised' and 'reflective' interviewing. Ethnographers do not have structured questions but may have a list of issues to be covered. Ethnographers may also change the mode of interviewing at different points in the same interview. The approach may be directive or non-directive depending on the function the questioning is intended to serve. Non-directive questions are designed as:

> Triggers that stimulate the interviewee into talking about a particular broad area.
>
> (Hammersley and Atkinson 1983: 113)

Such was the approach taken in this research. A number of topics were introduced into the conversation at different points, depending on the form and content of the particular interview. In the pilot the following areas of discussion were used:

A The probation officer was asked why particular people had been selected and paired.

B The probation officer was asked to describe the methods that were being used with that offender.

C The respondent was asked why a particular method had been chosen.

D The probation officer was asked to discuss the likely outcome of the probation intervention.

E The probation officer was asked to give an explanation for offending behaviour.

By raising these issues in the interview it was thought that probation officers would have the opportunity to link their perception of black and white offenders with practice. The subjects were also wide enough in scope to include a variety of perceptions.

In interviews following the pilot study it seemed appropriate to attempt to cover all the areas of discussion with at least two clients, one black and one white, in order to give a comparative dimension to the material. The interviews were recorded on cassette and transcribed. Although the process of transcription was long and laborious, it proved to be useful. The close inspection of the material demanded by transcription assisted the researcher in formulating initial ideas about the conceptual categories that could emerge from the data. There then followed a process whereby the tapes were played back while the transcript was being read. This process is mentioned widely in the literature.

> Much of the analysis process consists of listening to tapes while reading the transcripts, noting the topic numbers on to the transcripts, and marking particularly relevant passages. Listening to the tapes is important as it gives tone of voice, expression and emphasis that will be missing from the transcript. The researcher might then make note of initial ideas under various topic headings and proceed to gather data relating to each topic systematically, so developing hypotheses and assembling quotations from the transcripts to support them.
>
> (Walker 1985: 40)

The transcript was then returned to the probation officer to read and comment on. This important part of the methodology introduced respondent validation into the research. The need for respondent validation in qualitative research is widely debated in the literature. Schutz has argued that meanings must be reconstructed on the basis of memory and much social action operates at a subconscious level, leaving no memory traces. Social actors are 'well-placed informants' on their own actions. They are no more than that and their accounts must be analysed in the same way as any other data, with close attention being given to the possible threats to validity (Schutz 1964).

It became possible at this point to formulate categories of understanding. These led to questions of a more precise nature that could be tackled in the second interview.

Part c and b records on the offenders selected by the probation officer were then read. The initial problem experienced was that in some cases there were copious records dating back over a 10-year period. Much of the material seemed useful and relevant to the study and the temptation was to attempt to record it in full. This proved impossible, first because of the inordinate amount of time that this process would have taken, and second because of the overwhelming amount of documented material this would have given. The pilot study again revealed a need for selection. Although all these documents were read and particularly relevant points were noted, in one case from as far back as 1972, it was decided to restrict full recording of these documents to the last two years.

The second interview

At this point it was possible to put supplementary questions to the probation officer in the light of the research material gathered. The second interview also provided the opportunity for the respondent to add or to clarify points made in the first interview. There was a definable difference in the way in which the probation officer had responded in the first interview. The second phase created some unease as more specific points relating to practice were highlighted.

A note on categories

In the account given of the analysis of material, the term 'categories' is used frequently and it is necessary to clarify the meaning of the term. Lofland described two types of category in ethnography. 'Member-identified categories' refer to typifications that are employed by members themselves: that is, they are 'folk' categories, or in this case the categories of 'probation culture'. They are found in the 'situated vocabularies' of the given culture. 'Observer-identified categories' are types constructed by the observer (Lofland 1971). In this case the categories are both member-identified and observer-identified. Through the use of categories, this research seeks to test *a priori* propositions by coding and analysing all relevant data. In an attempt to do this a three-stage process of sequential analysis was utilised, derived from the work of Becker and Greer:

1 The selection and definition of problems, concepts and indices.

2 The check on frequency and distribution of phenomena.
3 The incorporation of individual findings into a model of organisation under study.

(Becker and Greer 1982: 241)

The analysis of material

Although the categories that emerged from the material gathered in interviews to some extent reflected the questions that had been asked, three dominant forms of explanation emerged from research materials. They were:

1 Explanations relating to offending behaviour.
2 Explanations relating to social-work methods.
3 Explanations relating to the personality of the offender.

Making sense of the data

After collecting material from all sources, a systematic form of analysis had to be devised. Each major category, offending, social-work methods and personality was examined separately. Large sheets of paper were used and categorised as shown below.

Po	b/w	code	Explanation SER	Explanation Interview 1	Explanation Interview 2	Explanation part c	Explanation part b

Explanations for offending behaviour

Offenders were identified by code. By using this method it was possible to examine the name of the probation officer and the code of the offender with the summarised explanations of offending from separate sources: interview 1, interview 2, records and social-enquiry reports. Probation officers from teams were analysed on the same sheets. The advantages of this method of analysis were numerous:

1 It enabled all the material to be examined in such a way that major emergent themes could be extracted and an holisic view of the material could be obtained at a glance
2 It facilitated the possibility of different orientations within teams to be examined.
3 It allowed a constant comparison to be made in relation to black

and white offenders. Simultaneously this method also allowed instant comparisons to be made between sources of material.

The constant comparative as described by Glaser and Strauss enables each segment of material to be examined in turn, and its relevance to one or more categories noted (Glaser and Strauss 1967). One segment is then compared with another, similarly categorised in order to map the data and to plot the emergent conceptual patterns (Hammersley and Atkinson 1983).

By using these summary diagrams it was possible to locate and then compare the content of the categories, putting together those that concerned the same topic or illustrated a particular conceptual theme. As Glaser and Strauss suggest, this process of comparison is one that generates concepts which relate to the dimensions and properties of the category. It also enables similarities and differences between categories to be compared with the way in which individual respondents construct reality. An independent assessor was also employed to compare emergent categories. Throughout the process of comparison, notes were made to record the findings of this comparative exercise.

After the initial themes had been recorded on the large sheets, by cutting the column horizontally it became possible to make comparisons at two levels:

A Between the pairings made by probation officers in the initial interviews.
B Between black and white individual offenders.

Comparisons were made at both a group and individual level. Working from left to right, each column was completed with reference to the research material. At this stage of the analysis the researcher was faced with a bewildering quantity of data. Further refinement and categorisation was required before any coherent meaning could be gained from the data. Each category was therefore divided into sub-categories, which facilitated a more detailed analysis.

Notes

INTRODUCTION

1 There is considerable debate in the probation service as to who is black. One group regard black people as being linked to each other by the common experience of oppression. Such a 'political' definition of black is being contested by other groups. Some argue that Asian history and culture is distinct from that of Africa and Europe. Some members of the Association of Black Probation Officers have broken away to form the National Association of Asian Probation Staff.

1 RACE, RACISM AND THE PROBATION SERVICE

1 Some might argue that the inter-relatedness of sentencing and probation practice makes such a distinction false. If probation research is not isolated at this point, it becomes impossible to separate research into probation practice from the plethora of data relating to other areas of the criminal justice system, e.g. policing and treatment in prison.
2 Quantitative research on the effects of anti-racist training needs to be conducted.

2 EXPLANATIONS FOR OFFENDING: THE PERCEPTIONS OF PROBATION OFFICERS

1 Italics introduced by the author to clarify which decision was being referred to by the officer.

3 SOCIAL-WORK PRACTICE WITH BLACK AND WHITE OFFENDERS

1 In Chapters 5 and 6, problems in utilising such a model will be discussed with specific reference to black offenders. The model is included at this stage to help illustrate the apparent lack of structure in practice, particularly with regard to evaluation.

2 Worral argues that some women are not definable within a professional discourse of femininity (nondescript women). In an attempt to avoid the 'gender contract' some women employ mechanisms that are interpreted by probation officers as devious or elusive. A similar phenomenon is being described in relation to conventional and unconventional explanations of white and black offending (Worral 1990).

4 LANGUAGE, POWER AND CONVENTION

1 The word 'developments' could be misleading. A lineal theoretical development from structuralism to post-structuralism is not being suggested. What is challenged is the notion that offending behaviour can be 'professionally' explained through an unbroken series of perceived causes and effects which can be communicated to sentencers. This chapter refers to the 'genealogical' exploration of official discourse (Foucault 1972; Rojek *et al.* 1988).

5 RACISM, ANTI-RACISM AND PROBATION POLICY

1 The Race Forum is a pressure group working against racism and is open to everyone in the service. The everyday business of the forum is conducted by an elected group.
2 The Criminal Justice Act 1991 received the Royal Assent on 25 July 1991. The main themes outlined in the White and Green Papers have been followed. After considerable lobbying from NAPO, the Society of Black Lawyers and the Association of Black Probation Officers, a clause was added to the Bill to place a duty on those administering the criminal justice system to 'avoid discriminating against any person on the basis of race, sex or any other improper ground'. A duty now falls upon the Home Office, under the Act, to publish regular statistics and information relating to discrimination in the criminal justice system.

Bibliography

ABSWAP (1983) *Black Children in Care: Evidence to the House of Commons Select Committee*, London: Association of Black Social Workers and Allied Professionals.

ACOP (1985) *Recruitment, Training, Racial Discrimination and the Probation Service*, London: Association of Chief Probation Officers.

Adorno, T. S., Frenkel-Brunswik, E., Levinson, D. J. and Sanforo, R. N. (1950) *The Authoritarian Personality*, London: Harper.

Ahmed, S. (1988) *Racism and Social Work Education*, unpublished lecture, National Institute of Social Work, London: 11 November.

Ahmed, S. (1991) 'Developing Anti-Racist Social Work Education Practice', in *Northern Curriculum Development Project – Setting the Context for Change*, Anti-Racist Social Work Education, London: Central Council for Education and Training in Social Work.

Ahmed, S. Cheetham, J. and Small, J. (eds) (1986) *Social Work with Black Children and their Families*, London: Batsford.

Allen, H. (1987) *Justice Unbalanced*, Milton Keynes: Open University Press.

Alsop, J. and Feldman, M. (1976) 'Personality and Anti-Social Behaviour', *British Journal of Criminology*, 16, 337–51.

Althusser, L. (1976) *Essays in Self-Criticism*, London: New Left Books.

Barthes, R. (1977) *Image, Music, Text*, London: Fontana.

Bean, P. (1976) *Rehabilitation and Deviance*, London: Routledge & Kegan Paul.

Becker, H. S. and Greer, B. (1982) 'Participant Observation: an analysis of qualitative field data', in Burgess, R. E. (ed.) *Field Research*, London: Allen & Unwin.

Bernstein, B. (1973) *Class Codes and Control, Volume 1, Theoretical Studies Towards a Sociology of Language*, St Albans, Paladin.

Bottoms, A. E. and McWilliams, W. (1979) 'A non-treatment paradigm for probation practice', *British Journal of Social Work*, 9, 159–202.

Bottoms, A. E. and Stellman, A. (1988) *Social Inquiry Reports*, Aldershot: Wildwood House.

Bourne, J. and Sivanandan, A. (1980) 'Cheerleaders and Ombudsmen: The Sociology of Race Relations in Britain', *Race and Class*, 21, 331–52.

Brake, M. (1980) *The Sociology of Youth Culture and Youth Subculture*, London: Routledge & Kegan Paul.

Brown, B. (1978) 'Behavioural Approaches to Child Care', *British Journal of Social Work*, 8, 313–26.

Burt, C. (1925) *The Young Delinquent*, London: University of London Press.

Campbell, H. (1980) 'Rastafari: Culture of Resistance', *Race and Class*, 22, (1), 1–23.

Carlen, P. (1976) *Magistrates Justice*, Oxford: Martin Robertson.

Carrington, B. and Denney, D. (1981) 'Young Rastafarians and the Probation Service', *Probation Journal*, 28 (4), 111–17.

Cashmore, E. (1979) *Rastaman: the Rastafarian Movement in England*, London: Allen & Unwin.

Cashmore, E. and Troyna, B. (1983) *Introduction to Race Relations*, London: Routledge & Kegan Paul.

CCETSW (1989) *Requirements and Regulations for the Dip SW*, (paper 30), London: Central Council for Education and Training in Social Work.

CCETSW (1991) *One Small Step Towards Racial Justice – the Teaching of Anti-Racism in Diploma in Social Work Programmes*, London: Central Council for Education and Training in Social Work.

CCPC (1983) *Probation: a Multi-Racial Approach*, London: Central Council of Probation Committees.

Cheetham, J. (1981) *Social Work Services for Ethnic Minorities, Report to the DHSS*, Oxford: Barnett House.

Cicourel, A. V. (1964) *Method and Measurement in Sociology*, New York: The Free Press.

Cicourel, A. V. (1968) *The Social Organisation of Juvenile Justice*, New York, John Wiley.

Community Relations Commission (1975) *Who Minds? A study of working mothers and childminding in ethnic minority communities*, London: Community Relation Council.

Coombe, V. and Little, A. (1986), *Race and Social Work*, London: Tavistock Publications.

Corrigan, P. and Leonard, P. (1978) *Social Work Practice Under Capitalism*, London: Macmillan.

Cousins, M. (1978) 'The Logic of Deconstruction', quoted in Worrall, A. (1990) *Offending Women*, London: Routledge.

Cox, O. C. (1948) *Caste, class and race: A study of social dynamics*, New York: Monthly Review Press.

Cox, O. C. (1976), *Race Relations: Elements and Dynamics*, Wayne State: Wayne State University Press.

CRE (1977) *A Home from Home? Some policy considerations on black children in residential care*, London: Commission for Racial Equality.

CRE (1990) *The Next Steps: What Government can do for racial equality in the 1990s*, London: Commission for Racial Equality.

Crowe, I. and Cove, J. (1984) 'Ethnic Minorities and the Courts', *Criminal Law Review*, 413–17.

Culler, J. (1983) *Barthes*, London: Fontana.

Davies, M. (1985) *The Essential Social Worker*, Aldershot: Gower.

Davies, M. (ed.) (1991) *The Sociology of Social Work*, London and New York: Routledge.

Day, P. (1981) *Social Work and Social Control*, London: Tavistock Publications.

De la Motta, K. (1984) *Blacks in the Criminal Justice System*, unpublished M. Sc. thesis, University of Aston.

Denney, D. (1976) *Rastafarians and the Probation Service*, unpublished M.A. thesis, University of Warwick.

Denney, D. (1983) 'Some Dominant Perspectives in the Literature Relating to Multi-Racial Social Work', *British Journal of Social Work*, 13, 149–74.

Denney, D. (1991) 'Anti-racism Probation Training and the Criminal Justice System', in CCETSW (1991) *One Small Step Towards Racial Justice, The Teaching of Anti-Racism in Diploma in Social Work Programmes*, London: Central Council for Education and Training in Social Work.

DHSS (1984) *Services for the under fives from ethnic minorities*, Department of Health and Social Security.

Dimbleby, R. and Burton, G. (1985) *More than Words, an introduction to communication*, London: Methuen.

Divine, D. (1991) 'The Value of Anti-Racism in Social Work Education and Training', in *Northern Curriculum Development Project: Setting the Context for Change*, London: Central Council for Education and Training in Social Work.

Dominelli, L. (1988) *Anti-Racist Social Work*, London and Basingstoke: Macmillan.

Downes, D. (1966) *The Delinquent Solution*, London: Routledge & Kegan Paul.

Ely, P. and Denney, D. (1987) *Social Work in a Multi-Racial Society*, Aldershot: Gower.

Erikson, G. D. (1966) *Childhood and Society*, Harmondsworth: Penguin.

Erikson, G. D. (1968) *Identity, Youth and Crisis*, London: Tavistock Publications.

Eyesenk, H. J. and Eyesenk, S. (1978) 'Psychopathy, Personality and Genetics', in Hare, R. and Schaeting, H. (eds) *Psychopathic Behaviour, approaches to research*, New York: Wiley.

Fevre, R. (1984) *Cheap Labour and Racial Discrimination*, Aldershot: Gower.

Fielding, N. (1984) *Probation Practice, Client Support and Social Control*, Aldershot: Gower.

Fletchman-Smith, B. (1984) 'Effects of Race on Adoption and Fostering', *International Journal of Social Psychiatry*, 1 (2), 121–8.

Folkard, M. S., Smith, D. E. and Smith, D. D. (1976) *Impact, Volume II*, Home Office Research Study No. 25, London: HMSO.

Foner, N. (1979) *Jamaica Farewell*, London: Routledge & Kegan Paul.

Foucault, M. (1972) *The Archaeology of Knowledge*, London: Routledge.

Francis, E. (1991) 'Racism and Mental Health: Some Concerns for Social Work', in *Northern Curriculum Development Project: Setting the Context for Change, Anti-Racist Social Work Education*, London: Central Council for Education and Training in Social Work Education.

Gardiner, J. D. (1982) 'Probation and After Care with Ethnic Minorities', unpublished M.Sc. thesis, Jesus College Oxford, quoted in Staplehurst, A. (1983) *Working with Young Afro-Caribbean Offenders*, Social Work Monograph, Norwich: University of East Anglia.

Genders, E. and Player, E. (1989) *Race Relations in Prisons*, Oxford: Oxford University Press.

Gibbons, J. (1984) 'Live Wires', *Social Work Today*, 15(24), 14–5.

Gilroy, P. (1987) *There Ain't No Black in the Union Jack*, London: Hutchinson.

Glaser, B. G. and Strauss, A. S. (1967) *The Discovery of Grounded Theory*, Chicago: Aldine.

Goldberg, E. M. (1977) 'Exploring the task centred casework model', *Social Work Today*, 9 (2), 9–14.

Goldberg, E. M. and Stanley, S. J. (1985) '*Task centred casework in a probation setting: part 2*', in Goldberg, E. M., Sinclair, I. and Gibbons, J. (eds) *Problems, Tasks and Outcomes: The Evaluation of Task Centred Casework in Three Settings*, London: Allen & Unwin.

Graef, R. (1989) *Talking Blues*, London: Collins.

Green, R. (1987) 'Racism and the offender: a probation response', in Harding, J. (ed.) *Probation and the Community*, London: Tavistock Publications.

Greenwood, V. (1982) 'The role and future of women's imprisonment', Noel Buxton Lecture (unpublished), in Walker, H. and Beaumont, B. (1985) *Working with Offenders*, London: Macmillan.

Guest, C. (1984) 'A comparative analysis of the career patterns of black and white offenders', unpublished M.Sc. thesis, Cranfield Institute of Technology.

Gunn, J. and Farrington, D. P. (eds) (1982) *Abnormal Offenders, Delinquency, and the Criminal Justice System*, Chichester: Wiley.

Hakim, C. (1987) *Research Design Strategies and Choices in the Design of Social Research*, London: Allen & Unwin.

Hall, S., Critcher, C., Jefferson, T., Clark, J. and Roberts, B. (1978) *Policing the Crisis: Mugging, the state and law and order*, London: Macmillan.

Hammersley, M. and Atkinson, P. (1983) *Ethnography, Principles in Practice*, London: Tavistock publications.

Haralambos, M. with Heald, R. (1980) *Sociology, Themes and Perspectives*, Slough: University Tutorial Press.

Hebdige, D. (1976) '*Reggae, Rastas, and Rudies,*' in Hall, S. and Jefferson, T. *Resistance Through Rituals*, London: Hutchinson.

Hedges, B. M. (1981) 'An Introduction to Social Research', in Walker, R. (ed.) *Applied Qualitative Research*, Aldershot: Gower.

Hedges, B. M. (1978) 'Sampling minority populations', in Wilson, M. (ed.) *Social and Educational Research in Action*, London: Longman.

Hepple, B. (1987) 'The Race Relations Acts and the Process of Change', *New Community*, 14, (1/2).

Hewitt, R. (1986) *White Talk, Black Talk*, Cambridge: Cambridge University Press.

Home Office (1976) *Rastafarianism/Ethiopian Orthodox Church*, Home Office Instruction 60/1976, London: Home Office.

Home Office (1977) *Probation and After-Care Service – Ethnic minorities*. Home Office Circular 113/1977, London: Home Office.

Home Office (1983) *Home Office Circular*, 17/1983, London: Home Office.

Home Office (1983) *Home Office Circular* 18/1983, London: Home Office.

Home Office (1986) 'Reconvictions of those given probation orders', in *Statistical Bulletin* 34/1986, London, Government Statistical Service.

Home Office (1988a) *Prison Statistics, England and Wales 1987*, Cmnd 547, London: HMSO.

Home Office (1988b) *Probation Service Policies on Race*, Home Office Circular 75/1988, London: Home Office.

Home Office (1989) *The Probation Service: Promoting Value for Money*, London: HMSO.

Home Office (1990a) *Crimes, Justice and Protecting the Public*, Cmnd 965, London: HMSO.

Home Office (1990b) *Supervision and Punishment in the Community*, Cmnd 966, London: HMSO.

Home Office (1990c) *Partnership in Dealing with Offenders in the Community*, London: Home Office.

Home Office (1991a) *Organising Supervision and Punishment in the Community – A Decision Document*, London: Home Office.

Home Office (1991b) *Discussion Document: Towards National Standards for Pre-Sentence Reports*. November. London: Home Office.

Hudson, B. (1989) 'Discrimination and disparity: the influence of race on sentencing', *New Community*, 16 (1), 21–32.

Husband, C. (1980) 'Culture, Context and Practice: racism in social work', in Bailey, P. and Brake, M. *Radical Social Work and Practice*, London: Edward Arnold.

Husband, C. (1991) '"Race", Conflictual Politics and Anti-Racist Social Work: Lessons from the past in the '90s', in *Northern Curriculum Development Project: Setting the Context for change, Anti-Racist Social Work Education*, London: Central Council for Education and Training in Social Work.

ILPAS (1982) *ILPAS in a Multi-Racial Society*, Inner London Probation and After-Care Service.

Jenkins, R. (1966) Speech given to Voluntary Liaison Committees, London: National Committee for Commonwealth Immigrants.

Jensen, A. R. (1969) 'How much can we boost IQ and scholastic achievement?' *Harvard Educational Review*, 39 (1), 1–123.

Jones, R. (1983) 'Justice, Social Work and Statutory Supervision', in Morris, A. and Giller, H. (eds) (1987) *Understanding Juvenile Justice*, London: Croom Helm.

King, M. and May, C. (1985) *Black Magistrates*, London: Cobden Trust.

Knowles, C. (1990) 'Black families and social services', in Cambridge, A. and Feuchtwang, S. (eds) *Anti-Racist Strategies*, Aldershot: Avebury.

Kirwin, K. (1985) 'Probation and Supervision', in Walker, H. and Beaumont, B. *Working with Offenders*, Basingstoke: Macmillan.

Lea, J. and Young, J. (1984) *What is to be done about law and order?*, Harmondsworth: Penguin.

Leicester City Council (1980) *Working party on ethnic minority youth.*

Leonard, P. (1975) 'Explanation and Education in Social Work', British Journal of Social Work, 5 (3), 325–33.

Levi-Strauss, C. (1973) *Tristes tropiques*, translated by Weightman, J. and Weightman, D., London: Cape.

Lodge, D. (1981) *Working with Structuralism*, London: Routledge.

Lofland, J. (1971) *Analysing Social Settings: a guide to qualitative research,* Belmont, California: Wadsworth.

Lowenthal, D. (1972) *West Indian Societies,* Oxford: Oxford University Press.

Mair, G. (1986) 'Ethnic Minorities and the Magistrates Court', *British Journal of Criminology*, 26 (2), 147–55.

May, T. (1991) *Probation: Politics, Policy and Practice*, Milton Keynes: Open University Press.

McConville, F. H. and Baldwin, J. (1982) 'The Influence of Race on Sentencing in England', *Criminal Law Review*, 652–8.

Merseyside Probation and After Care Committee (1976) 'Annual Report of the Chief Probation Officer', in Staplehurst, A. (1983) *Working with Young Afro-Caribbean Offenders*, Social Work Monograph, Norwich: University of East Anglia.

Mills, C. W. (1940) 'Situated Actions and Vocabularies of Motive', *American Sociological Review*, 5, 904–13.

Morris, A. and Giller, H. (1987) *Understanding Juvenile Justice*, London: Croom Helm.

Moxon, D. (1988) *Sentencing Practice in the Crown Court*, Home Office Research Study 103, London: HMSO.

NACRO (1986) *Black People in the Criminal Justice System.* London: National Association for the Care and Rehabilitation of Offenders.

NACRO (1987) *Juvenile Crime Briefing*, London: National Association for the Care and Resettlement of Offenders.

NACRO (1988) *The Electronic Monitoring of Offenders*, NACRO briefing, London: National Association for the Care and Resettlement of Offenders.

NACRO (1991a) *Race and Criminal Justice*, NACRO briefing, London: National Association for the Care and Resettlement of Offenders.

NACRO (1991b) *Black People's Experience of Criminal Justice*, London: National Association for the Care and Resettlement of Offenders.

Naik, D. (1991) 'An Examination of Social Work Education within an Anti-Racist Framework', in *National Curriculum Development Project, Setting the Context for Change, Anti-Racist Social Work Education*, London: Central Council for Education and Training in Social Work.

NAPO (1988) 'Racism, Representation, and the Criminal Justice System', *NAPO News*, No. 4, National Association of Probation Officers.

NAPO (1989) 'Black Probation Staff', (news item) *NAPO News*, September, London: National Association of Probation Officers.

NAPO (1990a) *The Response of the National Association of Probation Officers to the White Paper 'Crime, Justice and Protecting the Public'* Cmnd 965, London, National Association of Probation Officers.

NAPO (1990b) *The Response of the National Association of Probation Officers to the Green Paper 'Supervision and Punishment in the Community'*, London: National Association of Probation Officers.

NAPO (1991) *NAPO News*, May/June 1991, No. 30, London: National Association of Probation Officers.

Northern Curriculum Development Project (1991) *Setting the Context for Change – Anti-Racist Social Work Education*, London: Central Council for Education and Training in Social Work.

North East London Probation Service (1981) 'Annual Report', quoted in Staplehurst, A. (1983) *Working with Young Afro-Caribbean Offenders*, Social Work Monograph, Norwich: University of East Anglia.

Ollereanshaw, S. (1984) 'The Promotion of Employment Equity in Britain', in Glazer, N. and Young, K. (eds) *Ethnic Pluralism and Public Policy*, London: Heinemann.

Parnes, H. S. (1975) 'The National Longitudinal Surveys: new vistas for labour market research', *American Economic Review*, 65, 244–9.

Perry, F. G. (1979) *Reports for Criminal Courts*, Teddington, Owen Wells.

Phillpotts, G. J. O. and Lancucki, L. B. (1979) *Previous convictions, sentence, and reconvictions: a statistical study of a sample of 5,000 offenders convicted in January 1971*, Home Office Research Study No. 53, London: HMSO.

Pincus, A. and Minahan, A. (1973) *Social Work Practice and Method*, Illinois: Peacock Press.

Pinder, R. (1982) 'On what grounds negotiating justice with black clients', *Probation Journal*, 29(1), 19.

Pinder, R. (1983) 'Respecting differences: the ethnic challenge to social work practice', *Social Work Today*, Research and Practice series 14, 22.

Pinder, R. (1984) *Probation and ethnic diversity*, monograph, University of Leeds.

Pitts, J. (1984) 'Racism, Juvenile Justice and IT', *IT Mailing*, No. 17, July, 4–5, Leicester Youth Bureau.

Pitts, J. (1988) *The Politics of Juvenile Crime*, London: Sage.

Policy Studies Institute (1983) *Police and People in London*: London, Policy Studies Institute.

Popper, K. R. (1963) *Conjectures and Refutations*, London: Routledge & Kegan Paul.

Powdermaker, H. (1966) *Stranger and Friend: The Way of an Anthropologist*, New York: Norton.

Powell, M. (1985) 'Court Work', in Walker, H. and Beaumont, B., *Working with Offenders*, London: Macmillan.

Preston-Shoot, M. and Williams, J. (1987) 'Evaluating the Effectiveness of Practice', *Practice* 1(40).

Radical Statistics Group and Runnymede Trust (1980) *Britain's Black Population*, London: Heinemann Education.

Raynor, P. (1985) *Social Work, Justice and Control*, Oxford: Basil Blackwell.

Reid, W. and Epstein, L. (eds) (1977) *Task-Centred Practice*, Columbia: Columbia University Press.

Raynor, P. (1988) *Probation as an Alternative to Custody: a Case Study*, Aldershot: Gower.

Reiner, R. (1989) 'Race and criminal justice', *New Community*, 16(1), 5–21.

Rex, J. (1979) 'Black Militancy and Class Conflict' in Miles, R. and Philzaklea, A. (eds) *Racism and Political Action in Britain*, London: Routledge.

Rex, J. and Moore, R. (1967) *Community and Conflict*, Institute for Race Relations, Oxford, Oxford University Press.

Ridley, J. (1980) 'Implications of Rastafarianism in Young West Indians in Slough', B.A. dissertation, University of Reading, in Staplehurst, A. (1983) *Working with Young Afro-Caribbean Offenders*, Social Work Monograph, Norwich: University of East Anglia.

Rodger, J. J. (1991) 'Discourse Analysis and Social Relationships in Social Work', *British Journal of Social Work*, 21, 63–79.

Rogers, A. (1989) 'Young black people and the juvenile justice system', *New Community*, 16 (1).

Rosenhan, D. (1972) 'On being sane in insane places', *Science*, 179, 250–8, Routledge & Kegan Paul.

Rojek, C. and Collins, S. A. (1988) 'Contract or Con Trick Revisited: Comments on the reply by Corden and Preston-Shoot', *British Journal of Social Work*, 18, 611–22.

Rojek, C., Peacock, G. and Collins, S. (1988) *Social Work and Received Ideas*, London: Routledge.

Rutter, M. and Giller, H. (1983) *Juvenile Delinquency, Trends and Perspectives*, Harmondsworth: Penguin.

Saussure, F. de (1974) *Course in General Linguistics*, London: Fontana.

Schatzman, L. and Strauss, A. (1973) *Field Research: Strategies for a Natural Sociology*, Englewood Cliffs, NJ: Prentice Hall.

Schuessler, K. F. and Cressey, D. B. (1950) 'Personality Characteristics of Criminals', *American Journal of Sociology*, 55, 476–84.

Schutz, A. (1964) 'The Stranger: an essay in social psychology', in Schutz, A. (ed.) *Collected Papers*, Vol. II, The Hague: Martinus Nijhoff.

Scott, D. Stone, N., Simpson, P. and Falkingham, P. (eds) (1985) *Going Local in Probation? Case Studies in Community Practice*, University of East Anglia/University of Manchester.

Selden, R. (1989) *A Reader's Guide to Contemporary Literary Theory*, London: Harvester Wheatsheaf.

Shallice, A. and Gordon, P. (1990) *Black People, White Justice? Race and the Criminal Justice System*, London: Runnymede.

Sheldon, B. (1982) *Behaviour Modification*, London: Tavistock Publications.

Sibeon, R. (1991) 'The Construction of a Contemporary Sociology of Social Work', in Davies, M. (ed.) *The Sociology of Social Work*, London and New York: Routledge.

Sivanandan, A. (1981) 'From Resistance to Rebellion: Asian and Afro-Caribbean Struggles in Britain', *Race and Class*, 23 (2/3), 111–52.

Sivanandan, A. (1982) 'Race, Class and the State', in *A Different Hunger: Writings on Black Resistance*, London: Pluto Press.

Small, J. (1982) 'New Black Families', *Adoption and Fostering*, 6 (33).

Small, J. (1988) *Social Work, Education and Racism*, unpublished lecture at National Institute of Social Work, 11 November.

Smart, C. (1976) *Women, Crime and Criminology*, London: Routledge & Kegan Paul.
Smith, D. (1977) *Racial Disadvantage in Britain*, Harmondsworth: Penguin.
Smith, D. and Gray, J. (1983) *Police and People in London*, London: Policy Studies Institute/Heinemann.
Smith, G. (1980) *Social Need*, London: Routledge & Kegan Paul.
Solomos, J. (1988) *Black Youth, Racism and the State – the Policies of Ideology and Polity*, Cambridge: Cambridge University Press.
South East London Probation and After Care Service (1977) 'The West Indian Client', quoted in Staplehurst, A. (1983) *Working with Young Afro-Caribbean Offenders*, Social Work Monograph, Norwich: University of East Anglia.
Sproat, K. (1979) 'Using National Longitudinal Surveys to Track Young Workers', *Monthly Labour Review*, 102(10), 28–33.
Stanley, S. (1991) 'Studying Talk in Probation Interviews', in Davies, M. (ed.) *The Sociology of Social Work*, London: Routledge.
Staplehurst, A. (1983) *Working with Young Afro-Caribbean Offenders*, Social Work Monograph, Norwich: University of East Anglia.
Stevens, P. and Willis, C. (1979) *Race, Crime and Arrests*, Home Office Research Study, 58, London: HMSO.
Stubbs, P. (1985) 'The Employment of Black Social Workers: From 'Ethnic Sensitivity to Anti-Racism?', *Critical Social Policy* No. 12.
Sutton, A. (1983) 'Social Inquiry Reports to the Juvenile Courts', in Geach, H. and Szwed, E. (eds) *Providing Civil Justice for Children*, London: Edward Arnold.
Swingewood, A. (1977) *The Myth of Mass Culture*, London: Macmillan.
Taylor, W. (1981) *Probation and After Care in a Multi-Racial Society*, London: Commission for Racial Equality.
Troyna, B. and Smith, D. (1983) 'A Question of Numbers: Race Relations, Social Policy and the Media', in Golding, P. (ed.) *Mass Media and Social Policy*, Oxford: Martin Robertson.
Tutt, N. and Giller, H. (1985) 'Doing Justice to Great Expectations', *Community Care*, 17 January, 20–5.
Waldo, G. P. and Dinitz, R. (1967) 'Personality attributes of the criminal: an analysis of research studies, 1950–1965', *Journal of Crime and Delinquency*, 4, 185–202.
Walker, H. and Beaumont, B. (1981) *Probation Work: Critical Theory and Socialist Practice*, Oxford: Basil Blackwell.
Walker, H. and Beaumont, B. (1985) *Working with Offenders*, Basingstoke: Macmillan.
Walker, M. (1988) 'The Court Disposal of Young Males by Race in London, 1983', *British Journal of Criminology*, 28(4), 281–93.
Walker, R. (ed.) (1985) *Applied Qualitative Research*, Aldershot: Gower.
Wallcot, R. (1968) 'The West Indian in the casework setting', *Probation Journal*, 14(2).
Waters, R. (1988) 'Race and the Criminal Justice Process: Two Empirical Studies on Social Inquiry Reports and Ethnic Minority Defendants', *British Journal of Criminology*, 28(1), 82–94.

Waters, R. (1990) *Ethnic Minorities and the Criminal Justice System*, Aldershot: Avebury.

Webb, D. and Harris, R. (1984) 'Social workers and the supervision order: a case of occupational uncertainty', *British Journal of Social Work*, Vol. 14, 579–90.

West Midlands Probation Service (1984) *Race Forum*, publication leaflet, Birmingham, West Midlands Probation Service.

West Midlands Probation Service (1987) *Report on the Birmingham Court Social Enquiry Report Monitoring Exercise*, Birmingham: West Midlands Probation Service.

West Yorkshire Probation and After Care Service (1978) *Probation and After Care in West Yorkshire*, Sheffield: West Yorkshire Probation Service.

Whitehouse, P. (1980) *Probation in a Multi-Racial Context*, paper presented to the British Psychological Society Conference, Bradford University, 22–28 March.

Whitehouse, P. (1983) 'Race Bias and Social Enquiry Reports', *Probation Journal*, 30(2), 43–9.

Whittaker, J. (1974) *Social Treatment*, Chicago: Aldine.

Willis, A. (1986) 'Help and control in probation: an empirical assessment of probation practice', in Pointing, J. (ed.) *Alternatives to Custody*, Oxford: Basil Blackwell.

Willis, A. (1981) 'Effective Criminal Supervision – Towards New Standards and Goals'. Lecture to NAPO branch day conference at Darlington, in Raynor, P. (1985) *Social Work, Justice and Control*, Oxford: Blackwell.

Willis, C. (1983) 'The Use, Effectiveness and Impact of Police Stop and Search Powers', *Research and Planning Unit Paper 15*, London: HMSO.

Willis, P. (1977) *Learning to Labour*, London: Saxon House.

Wilmott, P. (1966) *Adolescent Boys of East London*, London: Routledge & Kegan Paul.

Worral, A. (1990) *Offending Women*, London: Routledge.

Wrong, D. H. (1961) 'The Oversocialised Conception of Man in Modern Sociology', *American Sociological Review*, 26, 184–93.

Index